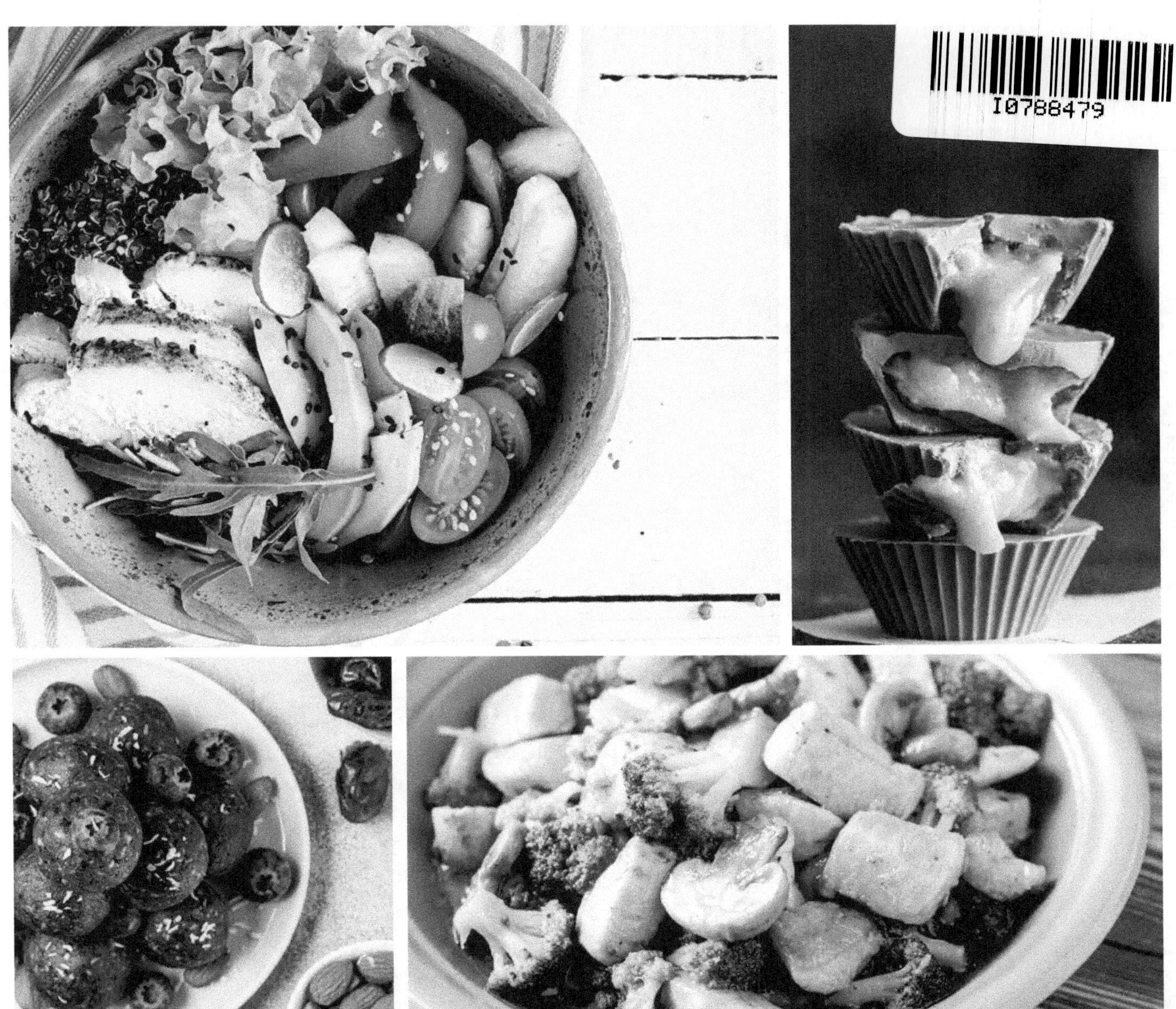

THE SIRTFOOD DIET COOKBOOK

SIMPLE, QUICK, AND DELICIOUS RECIPES FOR WEIGHT LOSS. WITH A COMPLETE HEALTHY MEAL PLAN TO BURN FAT AND ACTIVATE THE SKINNY GENE WHILE STILL ENJOYING YOUR FAVOURITE FOODS

ISABEL ADELE COOPER

BON APPETIT

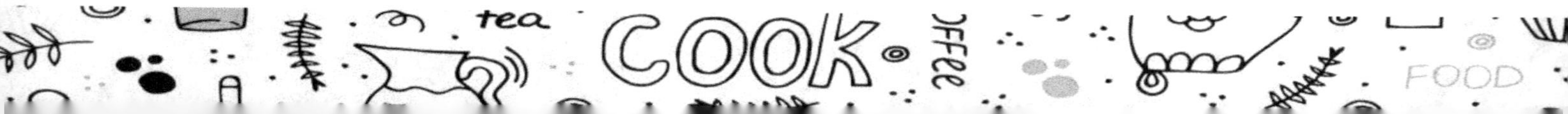
tea
COOK
COFFEE
FOOD

TABLE OF CONTENTS

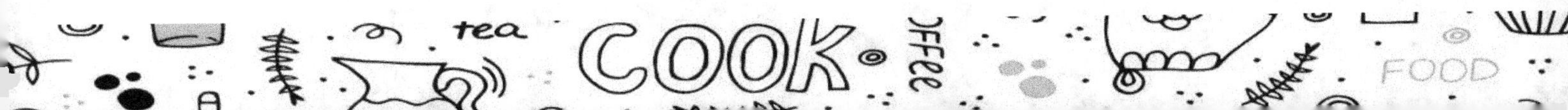

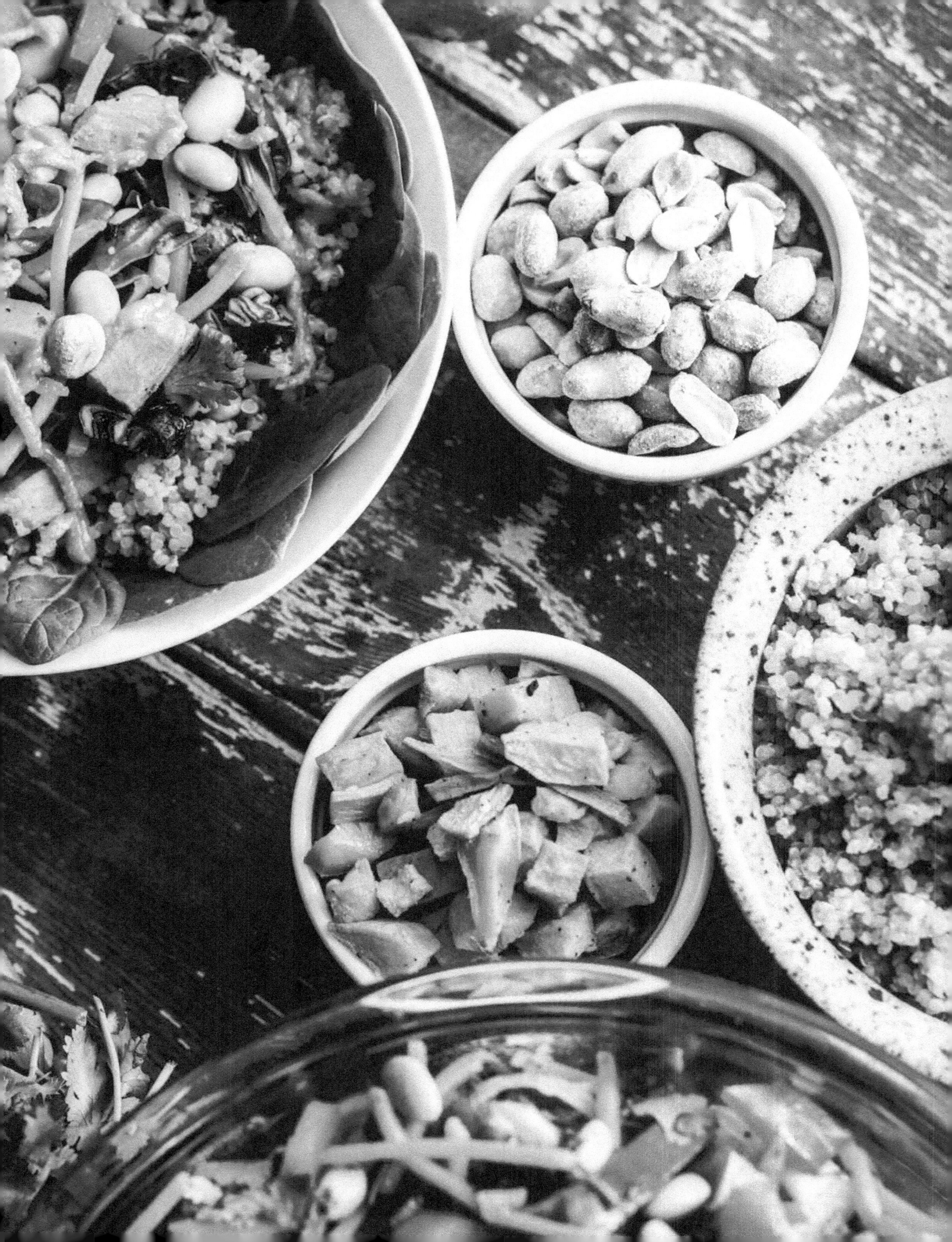

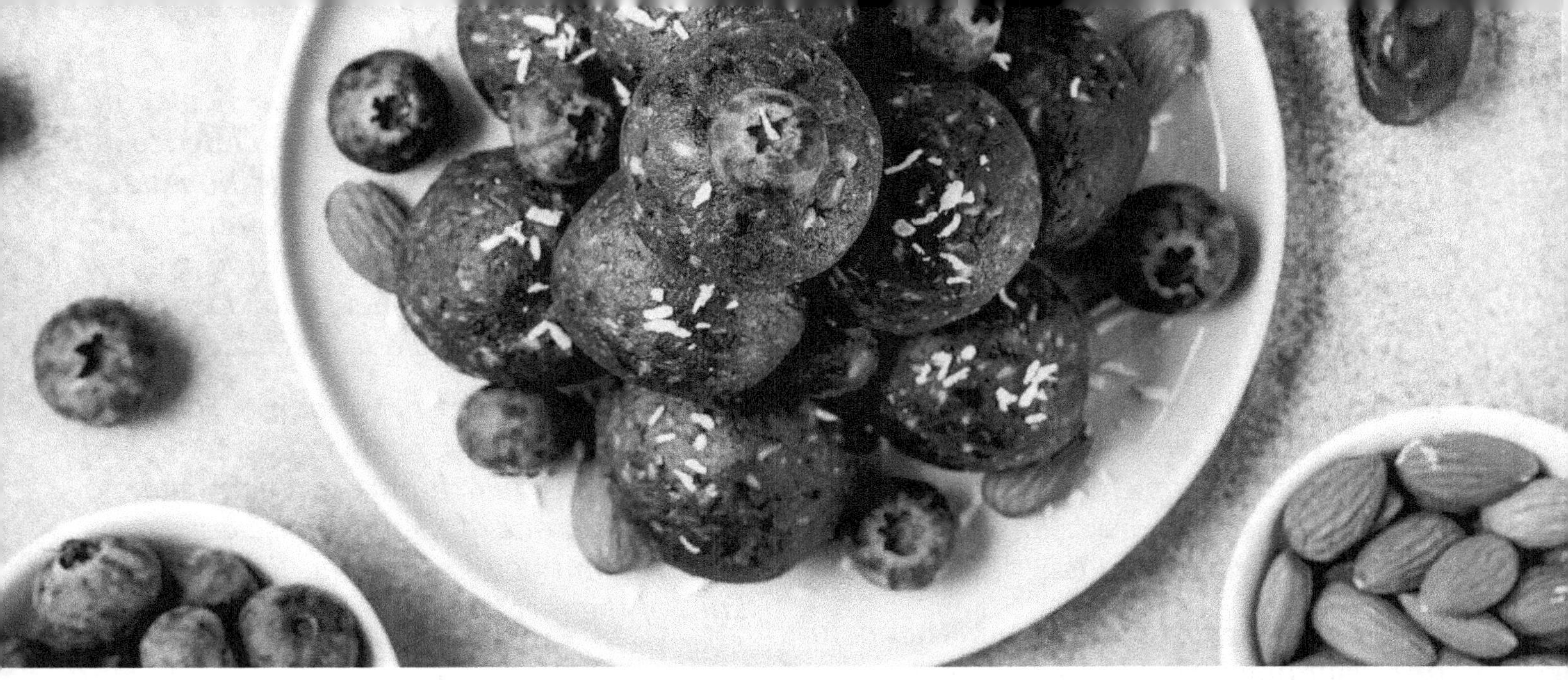

INTRODUCTION

On the off chance in which you don't comprehend why a specific eating routine works or expertise to adhere to it after the time for testing, you'll most likely abandon what you've realized. The other disappointing piece of most medicines is that such a large number of individuals will recover weight somewhat later, in light of the fact that they don't have the dubious thought of how or would incline toward not to keep carrying on with the new way of life. This eating routine is extraordinary.

In this book you will get comfortable with the sirtfood diet. These are particularly wealthy in supplements, prepared to make comparative fragile properties that move with fasting. These properties are called sirtuins and are viewed as answerable for absorption to influence our capacity to expend fat.

The Sirtfood Diet incorporates two phases.

Stage 1 guarantees the loss of 3.5 kg in 7 days and is the thing that makes the best outcomes. For the initial three days, you can eat an everyday cutoff of 1000 detached calories between three green juices and a healthy supper—everything relies upon Sirtfood. Starting with the fourth until the seventh day, calories will be at the rate of fifteen hundred. Two sirt juices and two in number Sirt meals are consolidated step by step.

Stage 2 is the upkeep stage and goes on for 14 days. During this period, the fundamental objective will be joining weight reduction. Regardless, it is conceivable to keep taking the structure by eating loads of Sirt supplements.

It is the ideal open door for you to turn out to be all the more amazingly crucial, vigorous, and fit with the goal that you can be a great individual. We think you value this book as we investigate the advantages of the Sirtfood

Diet!

While the famous low sugar diet is high in protein and permits just a moderate measure of starch, the Sirt Diet centers around sirtuins. These are impetuses in the body that shield the body's cells from uneasiness through their astounding development, particularly by decreasing the arrangement of free radicals. In an event that a large number of the supplements associated with serotonin creation are held by the body, it will likewise consume fat.

The favored position: Sirtuin activators are contained in a wide assortment of nourishments and refreshments, including exorbitant food sources, and therefore fortify a flimsy eating regimen that isn't amazingly restrictive. The principle undertaking of this eating regimen, in any case, is to devour a great deal of supplements, as it could be relied upon to be rich in these sirtuin activators.

Sirtuins fortify the safe structure, assist with working with bulk, and guarantees that cell absorption is diminished, hence the development procedure is decreased downwards, and you stay "more youthful." You simply must be all the more requesting with the assist you provide for others.

Sirtuins make you youthful and conservative, yet additionally unimaginable. The Sirtuin Diet Guarantee: In numerous weeks, you can lose as much as three pounds. In the event that you practice more and consume more calories, you can be a lot slimmer in this brief timeframe. Since the more muscle you have, the higher calories you consume. Supplements incited by sirtuin likewise decrease serious yearning assaults.

The most well-known woman who was supported by the Sirt diet is a totally genuine craftsman: Adele.

The Sirtfood diet should be wealthy in nourishments that contain a particular lift that actuates the body qualities related to fat mishaps and fat gathering. Additionally, a few people say they love it; given the route, there is a totally agreeable eating routine that has these welcome new upgrades (wine and chocolate), so you don't feel denied.

Any eating routine that requires solace of solace, supplements, for instance, wine and chocolate, is regularly hard to follow, making the Sirt Diet one of the most discussed diets of 2016, and you know why. Essentially in light of the fact that it is likely the primary food that doesn't restrict the utilization of wine and dull chocolate.

The Sirtfood diet has been touted as the essential eating routine that urges you to consolidate certain supplements rather than unquestionably decreasing your calorie admission.

BREAKFAST RECIPES

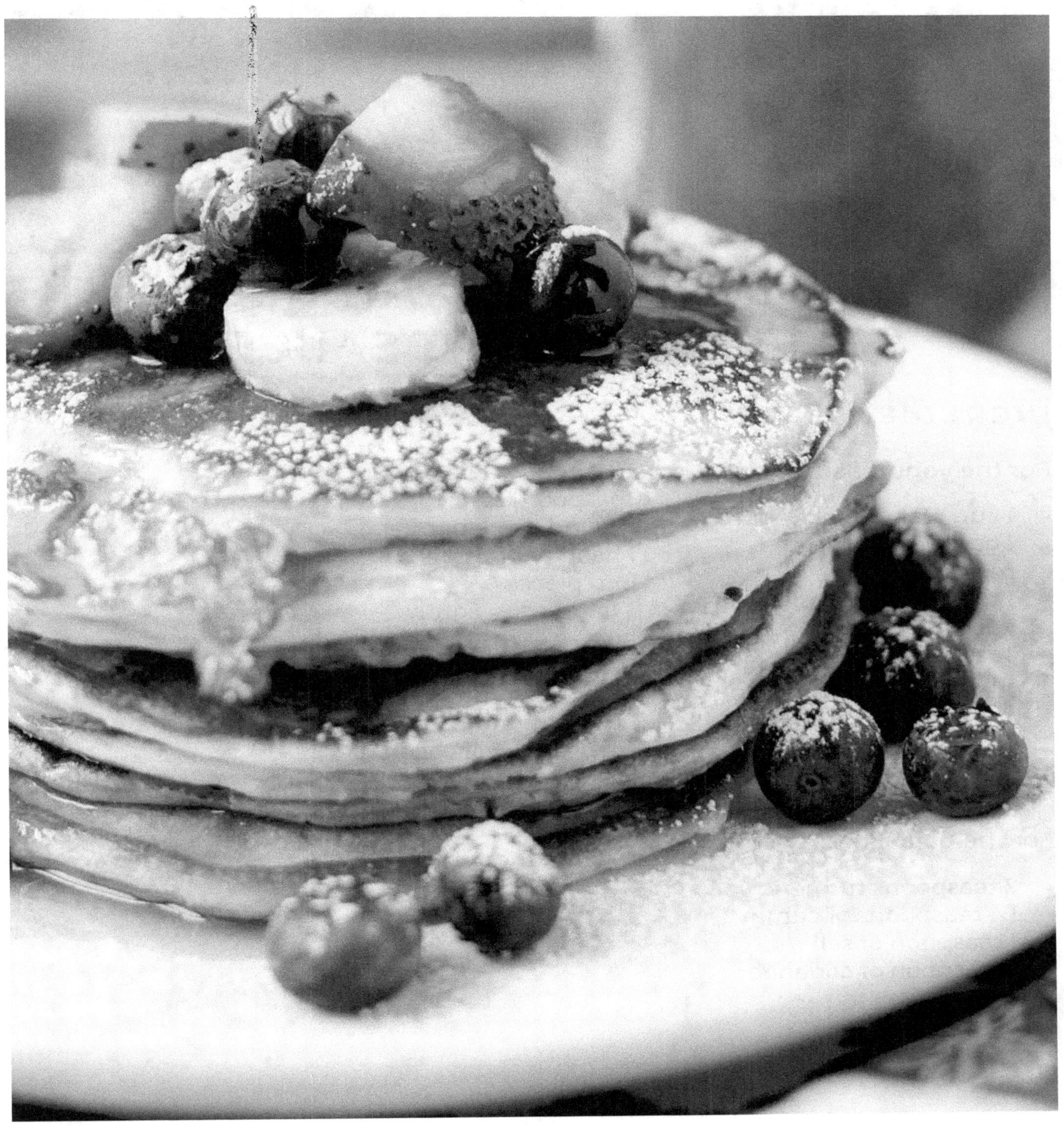

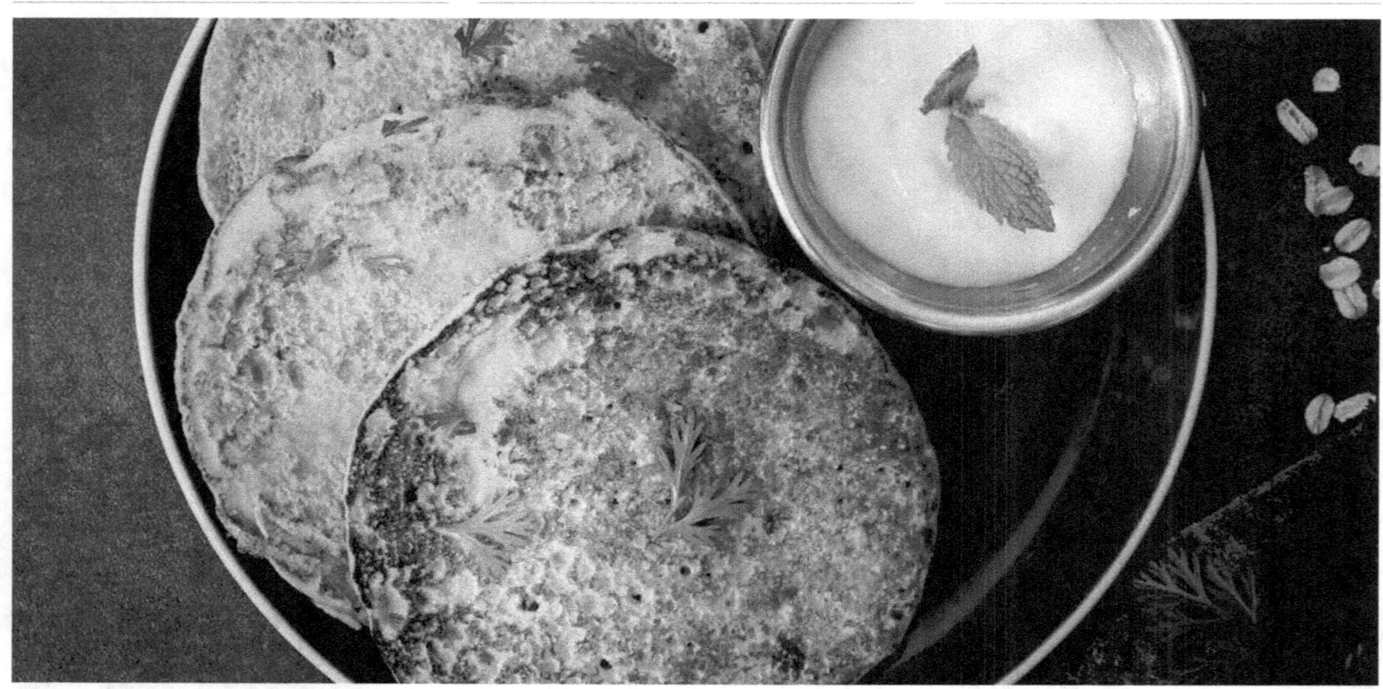

01. SAVORY TURMERIC PANCAKES WITH LEMON YOGURT SAUCE

INGREDIENTS

For the yogurt sauce:

- 1 cup plain Greek yogurt
- 1 garlic clove, minced meat
- 1 to 2 tablespoons lemon juice (1 lemon), to taste
- Teaspoon ground of turmeric
- 10 fresh mint leaves, minced meat
- 2 teaspoons grated lemon zest (from 1 lemon)

For the pancakes:

- 2 teaspoons turmeric
- 1½ teaspoons of cumin
- 1 teaspoon of salt
- 1 teaspoon of coriander
- Teaspoon garlic powder
- Teaspoon freshly ground black pepper
- 1 head of broccoli, cut into pieces
- 3 large eggs, lightly beaten
- 2 tablespoons of milk without almonds
- 1 cup almond flour
- 4 teaspoons of coconut oil

1. Make the yogurt sauce. Combine yogurt, garlic, lemon juice, turmeric, mint, and zest in a bowl. Try and season with more lemon juice, if necessary. Refrigerate or set aside until ready to serve.
2. Make the pancakes. In a small bowl, combine turmeric, cumin, salt, coriander, garlic, and pepper. Pour the broccoli in a food processor and beat until the pieces are separated into tiny pieces. Move the broccoli to a large bowl and add the eggs, almond milk, and almond flour. Add the spice mixture and mix well.
3. Heat 1 teaspoon of coconut oil in a nonstick skillet over medium-low heat. Pour the mixture from the dough cup into the pan.
4. Cook the pancake until tiny bubbles begin to appear on the surface and the bottom is golden, 2-3 minutes. Flip and cook the pancake for another 2 to 3 minutes. To retain heat, transfer cooked pancakes to a baking sheet and place in a 200°F oven.
5. Continue making the other 3 pancakes, using the remaining oil and whisking.

Nutritions: *Calories 234, Protein 43 g, Fat 9 g, Carbohydrate 44 g*

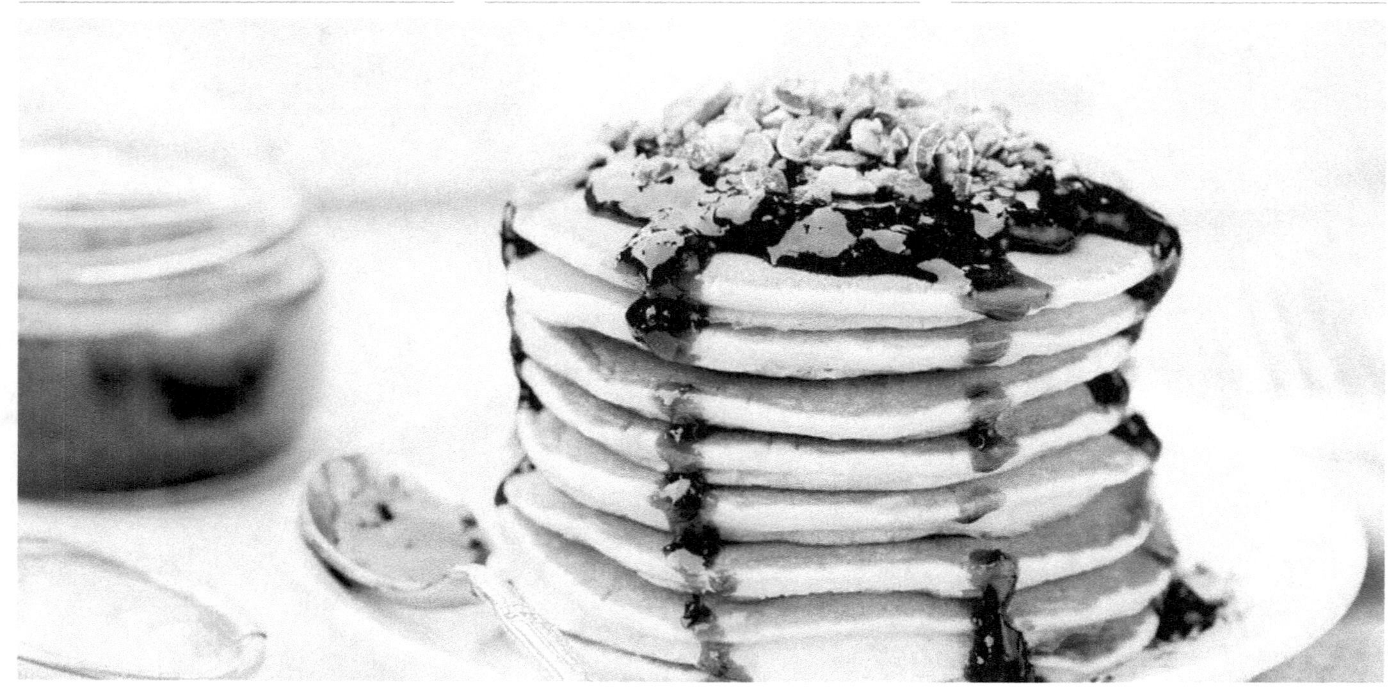

2. PANCAKES WITH APPLES AND BLACKCURRANTS

INGREDIENTS

- 2 apples cut into small chunks
- 2 cups of quick cooking oats
- 1 cup flour of your choice
- 1 teaspoon baking powder
- 2 tablespoons raw sugar, coconut sugar, or 2 tablespoons honey that is warm and easy to distribute
- 2 egg whites
- 1 ¼ cups of milk (or soy/rice/coconut)
- 2 teaspoon extra virgin olive oil
- A dash of salt

For the berry topping:

- 1 cup blackcurrants, washed and stalks removed
- 3 tablespoons water (may use less)
- 2 tablespoons sugar (see above for types)butter

DIRECTIONS

1. Place the ingredients for the topping in a small pot simmer, stirring frequently for about 10 minutes until it cooks down and the juices are released.
2. Take the dry ingredients and mix in a bowl. After, add the apples and the milk a bit at a time (you may not use it all), until it is a batter. Stiffly whisk the egg whites and then gently mix them into the pancake batter. Set aside in the refrigerator.
3. Pour a one quarter of the oil onto a flat pan or flat griddle, and when it is hot; pour some of the batter into it in a pancake shape. When the pancakes start to have golden brown edges and form air bubbles, they may be ready to be gently flipped.
4. Test to be sure the bottom can be easily removed away from the pan before actually flipping. Repeat for the next three pancakes. Top each pancake with the berries.

Nutritions: *Calories 377, Protein 9 g, Carbs 3 g, Fiber 8 g*

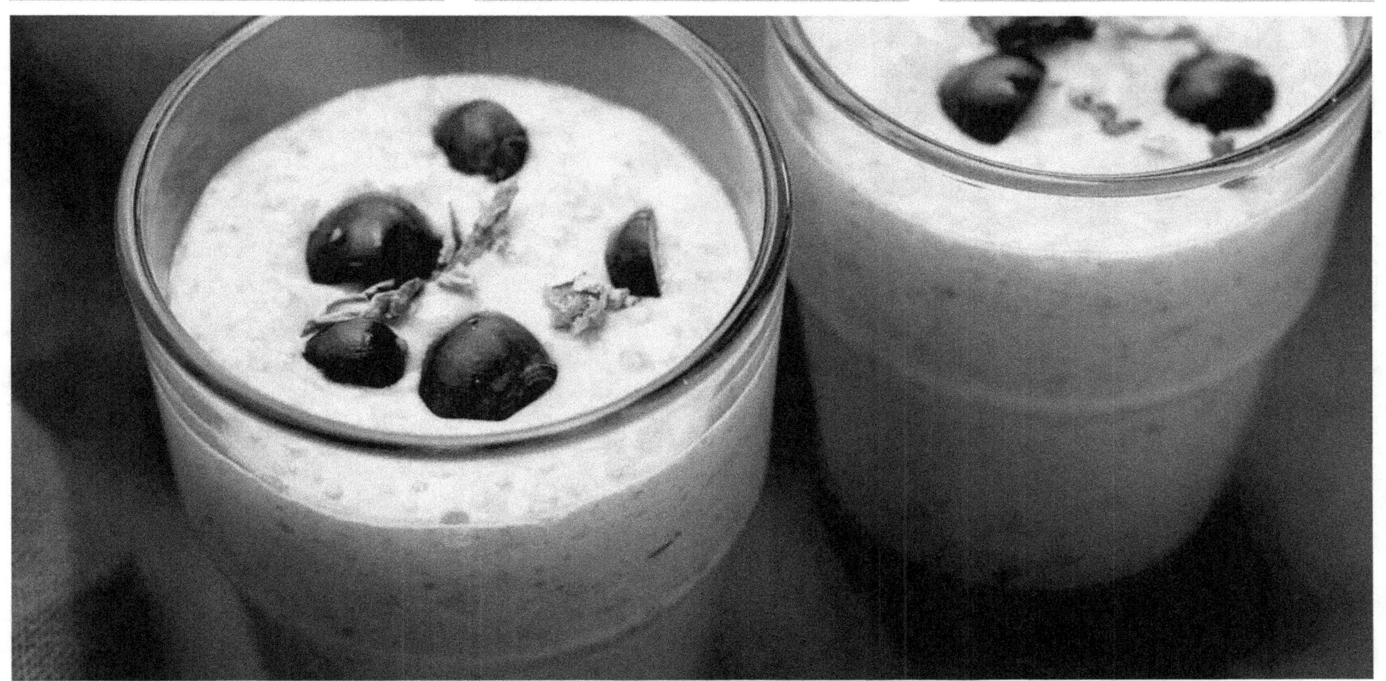

3. BLACK FOREST SMOOTHIE

INGREDIENTS

- 100g (3½ ounces) frozen cherries
- 25g (1 ounce) kale
- 1 medjool date
- 1 tablespoon cocoa powder
- 2 teaspoons chia seeds
- 200mls (7 fluid ounces) milk or soya milk

DIRECTIONS

1. Pour all your ingredients into a blender.
2. Process until smooth and creamy.

Nutritions: *Calories 233, Protein 23 g, Fat 15 g*

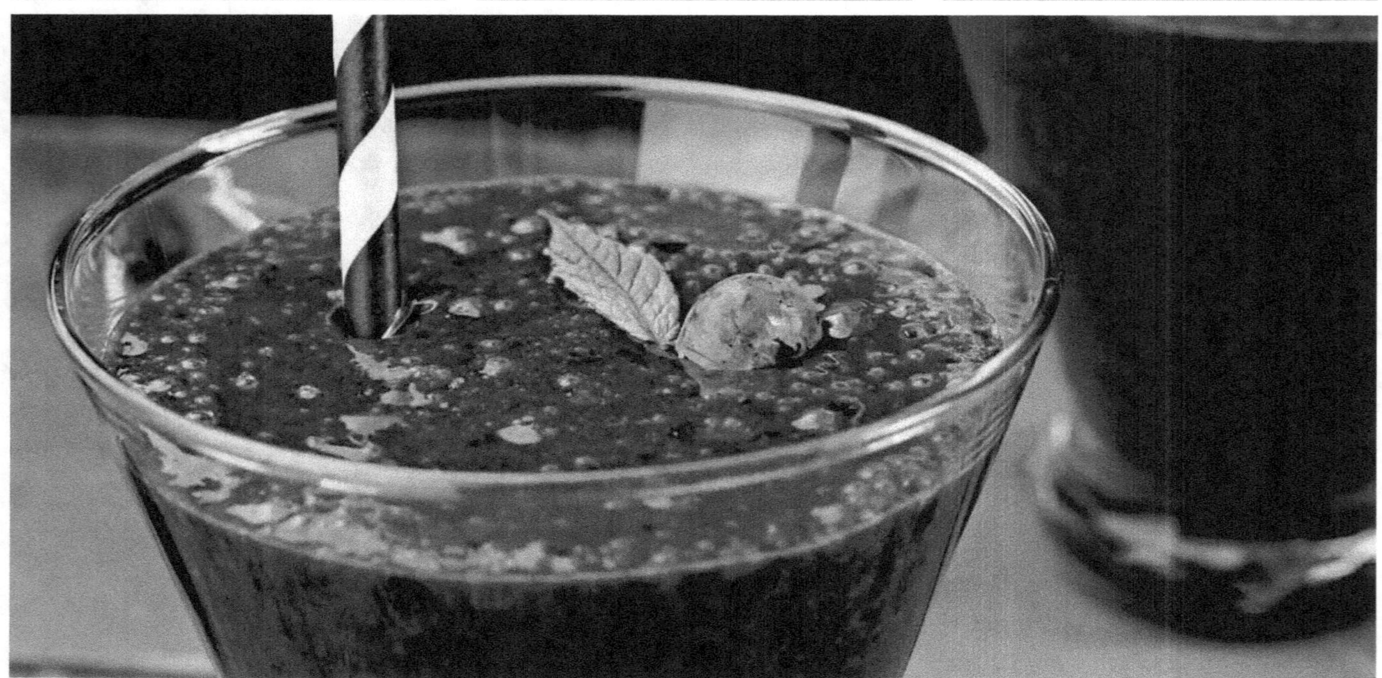

4. KALE AND BLACKCURRANT SMOOTHIE

INGREDIENTS

- 2 teaspoons honey
- 1 cup freshly made matcha green tea
- 10 baby kale leaves, stalks removed
- 1 ripe banana
- 40g blackcurrants, washed and stalks removed
- 6 ice cubes

DIRECTIONS

1. Mix the honey in the hot green tea until it dissolves.
2. Put all the ingredients together in a blender until smooth. Serve immediately.

Nutritions: *Calories 125, Sugar 6 g, Vitamin A and K*

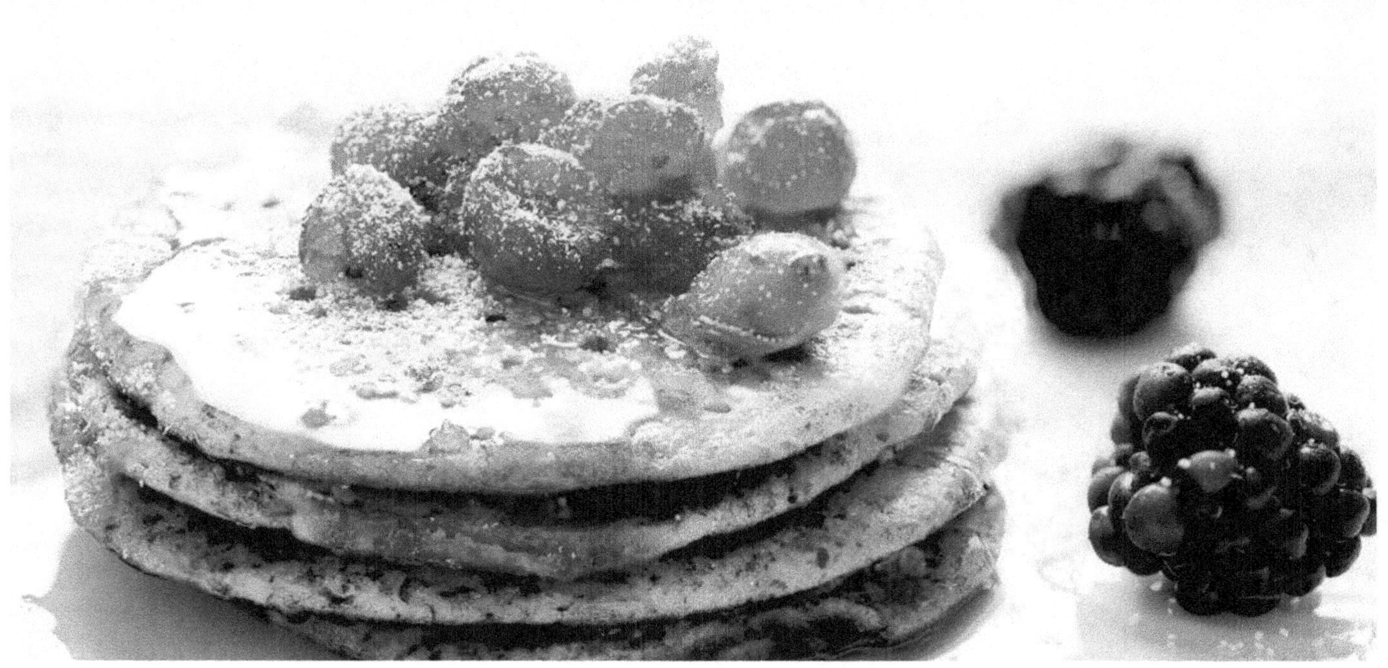

5. BUCKWHEAT PANCAKES

INGREDIENTS

- 1 cup coconut milk
- 2 teaspoons apple cider vinegar
- 1 cup buckwheat flour
- 2 tablespoons ground flax seed
- 1 tablespoon baking powder
- ¼ teaspoon sea salt
- ¼ cup maple syrup
- 1 teaspoon vanilla extract
- 1 tablespoon coconut oil

DIRECTIONS

1. Mix together the coconut milk and vinegar in a medium bowl. Set aside.
2. In a large bowl, mix together the flour, flax seed, baking powder, and salt.
3. Add the coconut milk mixture, maple syrup, and vanilla extract. Beat until well combined.
4. In a nonstick skillet, melt coconut oil over medium heat.
5. Pour about 1/3 cup of the coconut milk mixture and spread in an even circle.
6. Cook for about 1-2 minutes.
7. Flip and cook for an additional 1 minute, then remove from the pan.
8. Repeat with the remaining mixture.
9. Serve warm.

Nutritions: *Calories 345, Carbohydrate 76 g, Fat 3 g*

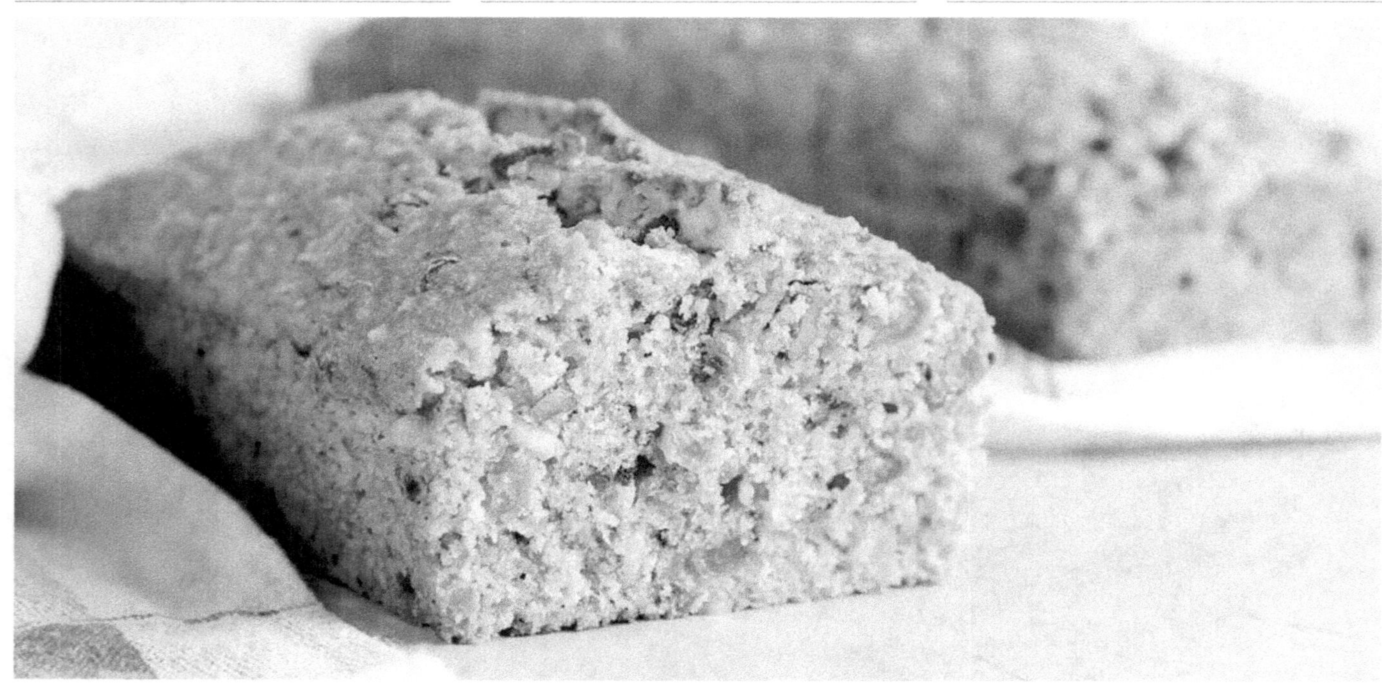

6. VEGETABLE & NUT LOAF

INGREDIENTS

- 175g (6 ounces) mushrooms, finely chopped
- 100g (3½ ounces) haricot beans
- 100g (3½ ounces) walnuts, finely chopped
- 100g (3½ ounces) peanuts, finely chopped
- 1 carrot, finely chopped
- 3 sticks celery, finely chopped
- 1 bird's-eye chili, finely chopped
- 1 red onion, finely chopped
- 1 egg, beaten
- 2 cloves of garlic, chopped
- 2 tablespoons olive oil
- 2 teaspoons turmeric powder
- 2 tablespoons soy sauce
- 4 tablespoons fresh parsley, chopped
- 100mls (3½ fluid ounces) water
- 60mls (2 fluid ounces) red wine

Nutritions: *Calories 312, Vitamin K, Carbohydrate 32 g*

DIRECTIONS

1. Heat your oil in a pan and add the garlic, chili, carrot, celery, onion, mushrooms and turmeric. Cook for 5 minutes. Place the haricot beans in a bowl and stir in the nuts, vegetables, soy sauce, egg, parsley, red wine and water.
2. Grease and line a large loaf tin with grease-proof paper. Place the mixture into the loaf tin, cover with foil and bake in the oven at 190°C/375°F for 60-90 minutes. Let it stand for 10 minutes, then turn onto a serving plate.

7. DATES & PARMA HAM

INGREDIENTS

- 12 medjool dates
- 2 slices of Parma ham cut into strips

DIRECTIONS

1. Wrap each date with a strip of Parma ham; it can be served hot or cold.

Nutritions: *Calories 321, Protein 22 g, Fat 8 g*

8. BRAISED CELERY

INGREDIENTS

- 250g (9 ounces) celery, chopped
- 100mls (3½ fluid ounces) warm vegetable stock (broth)
- 1 red onion, chopped
- 1 clove of garlic, crushed
- 1 tablespoon fresh parsley, chopped
- 25g (1 ounce) butter
- Sea salt and freshly ground black pepper

DIRECTIONS

1. Place the celery, onion, stock (broth) and garlic into a saucepan and bring it to the boil, reduce the heat and simmer for 10 minutes.
2. Stir in the parsley and butter and season with salt and pepper. Serve as an accompaniment to roast meat dishes.

Nutritions: *Calories 233, Carbohydrate 45 g, Sugar 6 g*

9. KALE & BROCCOLI SMOOTHIE

INGREDIENTS

- 1 cup of peeled and chopped roughly cucumber
- 2 cups fresh baby kale
- 1 cup frozen broccoli
- 1 tablespoon fresh lime juice
- 1½ cup unsweetened almond milk
- ½ cup ice, crushed

DIRECTIONS

1. Add all ingredients in a high-power blender and pulse until smooth.
2. Pour the smoothie into two glasses and serve immediately.

Nutritions: *Calories 123, Protein 65 g, Vitamin 12 g*

PREPARATION: 10 MIN   COOKING: 7 MIN   SERVES: 4

10. SALMON & KALE OMELET

INGREDIENTS

- 6 eggs
- 2 tablespoons unsweetened almond milk
- Salt and ground black pepper, as required
- 2 tablespoons olive oil
- 4 ounces smoked salmon, cut into bite-sized chunks
- 2 cups fresh kale, tough ribs removed and chopped finely
- 4 scallions, chopped finely

DIRECTIONS

1. In a bowl, place the eggs, coconut milk, salt and black pepper and beat well. Set aside.
2. In a nonstick wok, heat the oil over medium heat.
3. Place the egg mixture evenly and cook for about 30 seconds without stirring.
4. Place the salmon kale and scallions on top of the egg mixture evenly.
5. Now, adjust the heat to low and cook, covered for about 4-5 minutes or until omelet is done completely.
6. Uncover the wok and cook for about 1 minute.
7. Carefully, transfer the omelet onto a serving plate and serve.

Nutritions: *Calories 213, Protein 51 g, Fat 7 g*

11. KALE SCRAMBLE

INGREDIENTS

- 4 eggs
- 1/8 teaspoon ground turmeric
- Salt and ground black pepper, as required
- 1 tablespoon water
- 2 teaspoons olive oil
- 1 cup fresh kale, tough ribs removed and chopped

DIRECTIONS

1. In a bowl, place eggs, turmeric, salt, black pepper and water. With a whisk, beat until foamy.
2. Heat the oil over average heat in a wok.
3. Stir in the egg mixture and immediately reduce the heat to medium-low.
4. Cook for about 1-2 minutes, stirring frequently.
5. Stir in the kale and cook for about 3-4 minutes just like before.
6. Remove the wok from heat and serve immediately.

Nutritions: *Calories 356, Protein 78 g, Fat 6 g*

PREPARATION: 10 MIN   COOKING: 20 MIN   SERVES: 2

12. SCRAMBLE EGGS WITH MUSHROOMS

INGREDIENTS

- 2 eggs
- 1 teaspoon ground turmeric
- 1 teaspoon mild curry powder
- 1 teaspoon extra virgin olive oil
- 100g mushrooms, thinly sliced
- 5g parsley, finely chopped

DIRECTIONS

1. Heat the oil in a frying pan over medium heat, and fry the chili and mushrooms for 2–3 minutes until they have started to brown.
2. Mix the spices and add to the eggs. Top with the parsley.

Nutritions: *Calories 333, Protein 66 g, Fat 9 g, Carbohydrate 98 g*

13. GREEN TEA SMOOTHIE

INGREDIENTS

- 2 teaspoons of honey
- 250ml of milk
- 2 teaspoons of matcha green tea powder
- 6 ice cubes
- ½ teaspoon of vanilla bean paste (not extract) or a scrape of the seeds from the vanilla pod
- 2 ripe bananas

DIRECTIONS

1. Get a blender; place all the ingredients in the blender and run until you achieve a desired consistency.
2. Serve into two glasses and enjoy.

Nutritions: *Calories 155, Protein 32 g, Carbs 9 g, Fat 3 g*

14. PINK OMELETS

INGREDIENTS

- 2 eggs
- 100 g smoked salmon, sliced
- 20 g capers
- 20 g rocket, chopped
- 10g parsley, chopped
- 1 teaspoon olive oil

DIRECTIONS

1. Get a bowl, crack the eggs into the bowl and mix well with salmon, capers, rocket and parsley.
2. Heat the olive oil in a pan; add the egg mixture and, using a spatula or fish slice, move the mixture around the pan. Reduce the heat and let the omelet cook through.

Nutritions: *Calories 232, Fat 15 g, Protein 79 g*

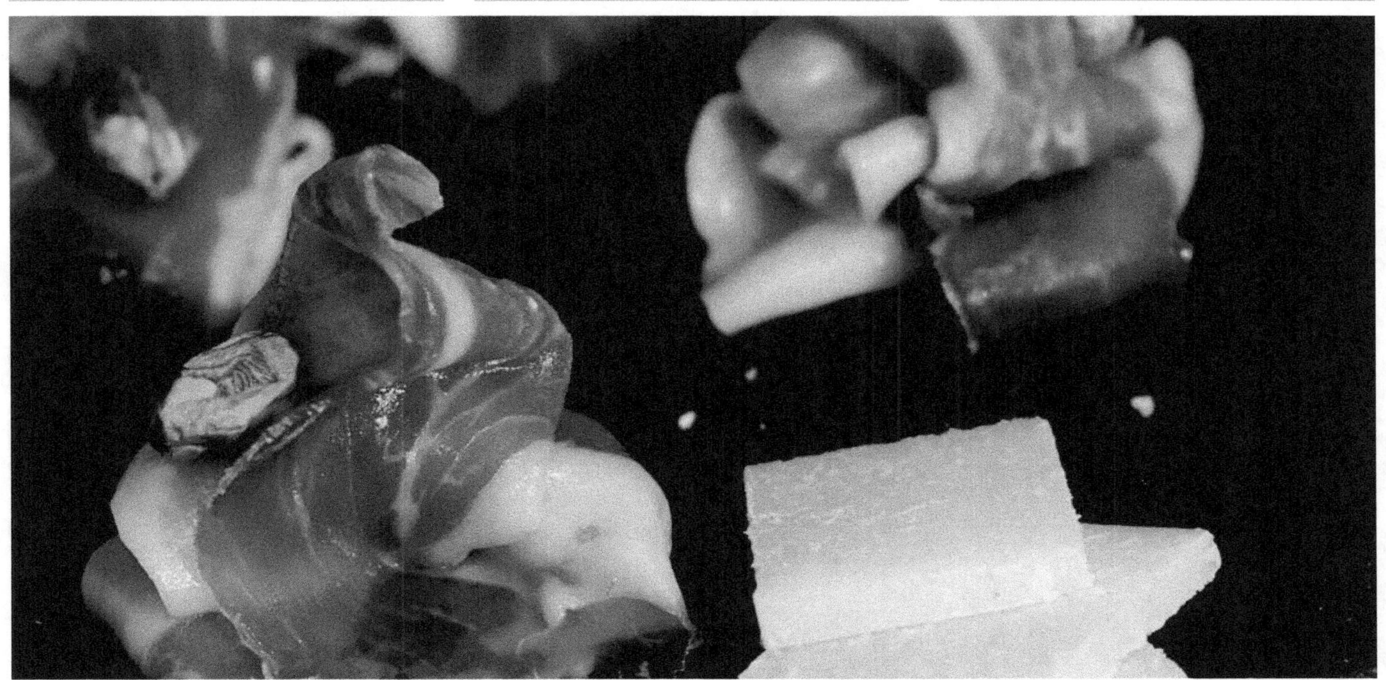

15. RED CHICORY
& STILTON CHEESE BOATS

INGREDIENTS

- 200g (7 ounces) Stilton cheese, crumbled
- 200g (7 ounces) red chicory leaves (or if unavailable, use yellow)
- 2 tablespoons fresh parsley, chopped
- 1 tablespoon olive oil

DIRECTIONS

1. Place the red chicory leaves onto a baking sheet. Sprinkle with cheese and drizzle with olive oil in the leaves.
2. Put them under a heated grill (broiler) for around 4 minutes until the cheese has melted.
3. Sprinkle with chopped parsley and serve immediately.

Nutritions: *Calories 651, Fat 25 g, Protein 23 g*

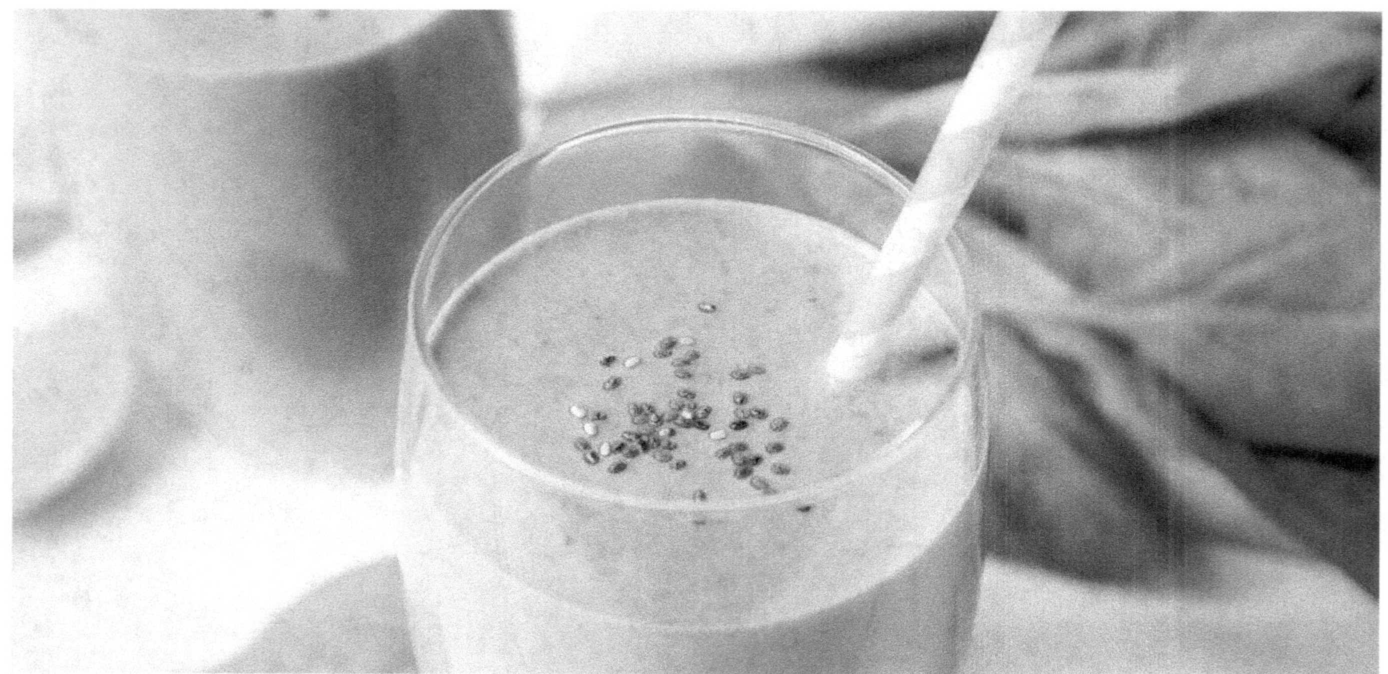

16. MATCHA GREEN JUICE

INGREDIENTS

- 5 ounces fresh kale
- 2 ounces fresh arugula
- ¼ cup fresh parsley
- 4 celery stalks
- 1 green apple, cored and chopped
- 1 (1-inch) piece fresh ginger, peeled
- 1 lemon, peeled
- ½ teaspoon matcha green tea

DIRECTIONS

1. Add all ingredients into a juicer and extract the juice according to the manufacturer's method.
2. Pour into 2 glasses and serve immediately.

Nutritions: *Calories 113, Total Fat 0.6 g, Saturated Fat 0.1 g, Cholesterol 0 mg, Sodium 71 mg, Total Carbs 26.71 g, Fiber 5.3 g Sugar 12.9 g, Protein 3.8 g*

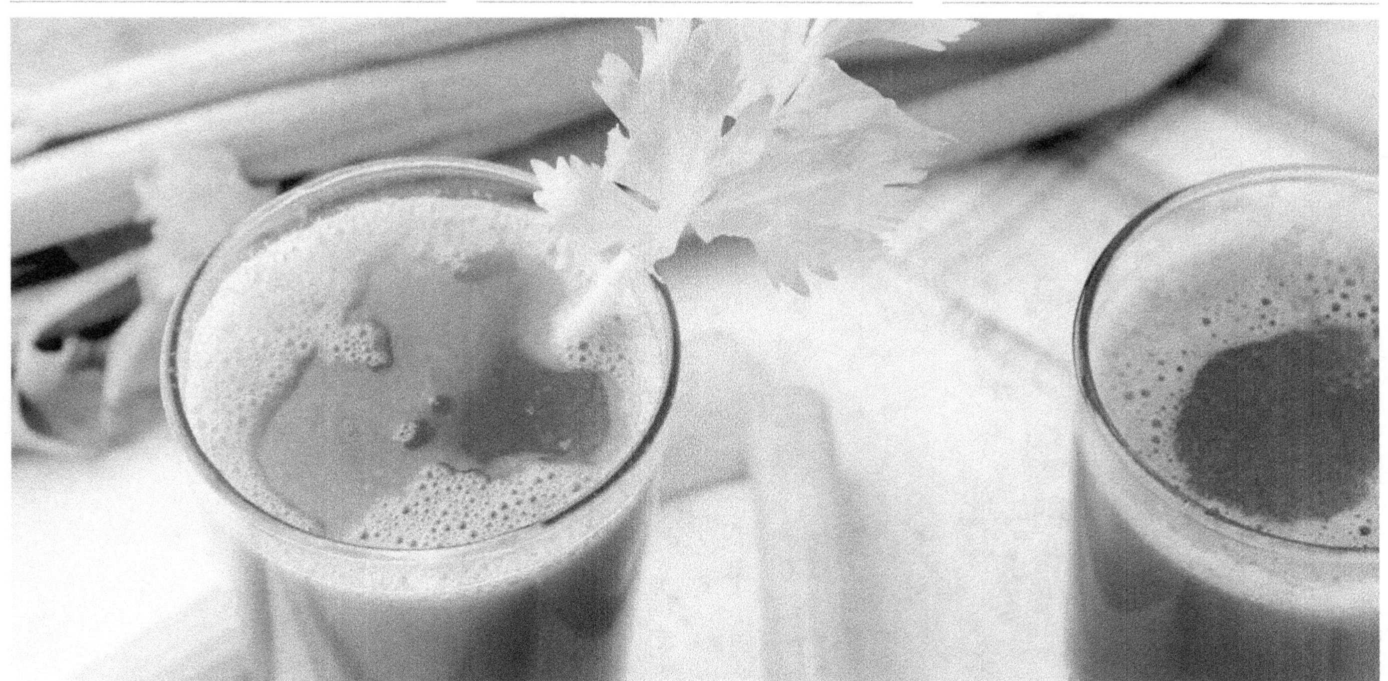

17. CELERY JUICE

INGREDIENTS

- 8 celery stalks with leaves
- 2 tablespoons fresh ginger, peeled
- 1 lemon, peeled
- ½ cup filtered water
- Pinch of salt

DIRECTIONS

1. Get a blender, place all the ingredients in the blender and pulse until well combined.
2. Through a fine mesh strainer, strain the juice and transfer into 2 glasses.
3. Serve immediately.

Nutritions: *Calories 32, Total Fat 0.5 g, Saturated Fat 0.1 g, Cholesterol 0 mg Sodium 134 mg, Total Carbs 6.5 g, Fiber 2 g, Sugar 1.3 g, Protein 1 g*

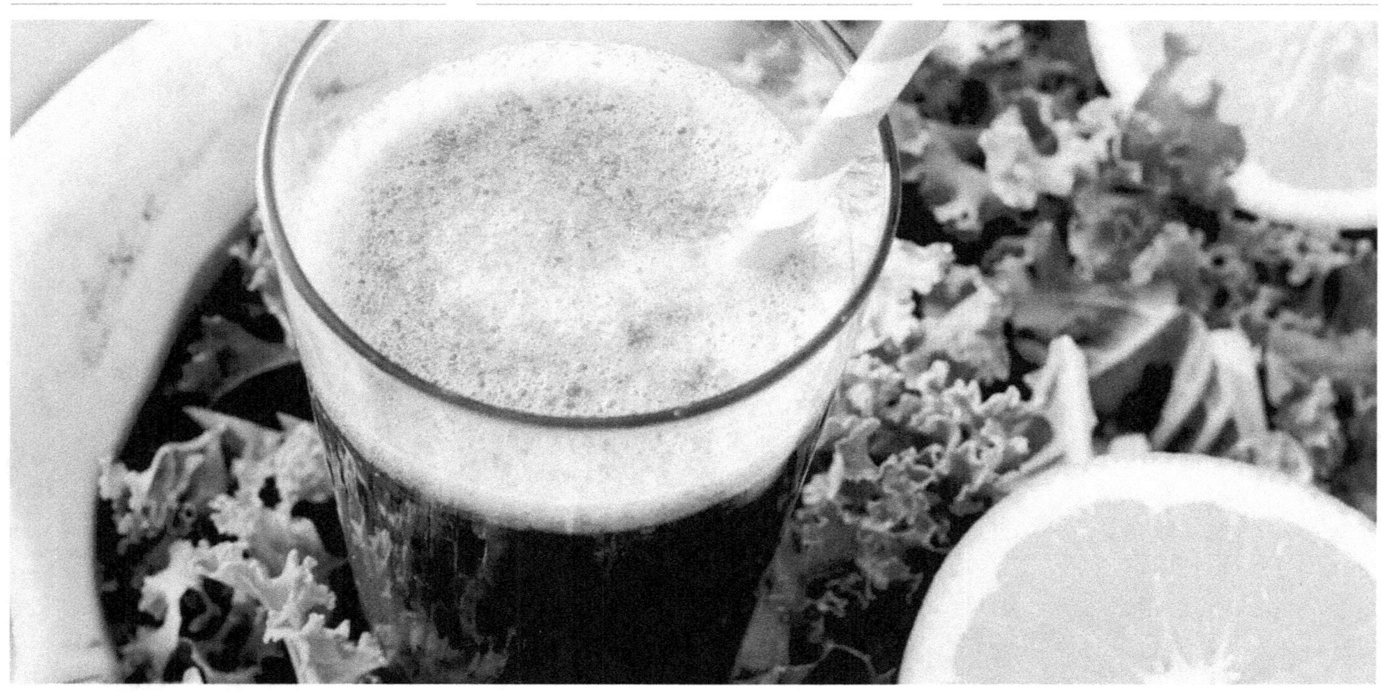

18. KALE & ORANGE JUICE

INGREDIENTS

- 5 large oranges, peeled and sectioned
- 2 bunches fresh kale

DIRECTIONS

1. Add all ingredients into a juicer and extract the juice according to the manufacturer's method.
2. Pour into 2 glasses and serve immediately.

Nutritions: *Calories 315, Total Fat 0.6 g, Saturated Fat 0.1 g, Cholesterol 0mg, Sodium 87 mg, Total Carbs 75.1 g, Fiber 14 g, Sugar 4.3 g, Protein 10.3 g*

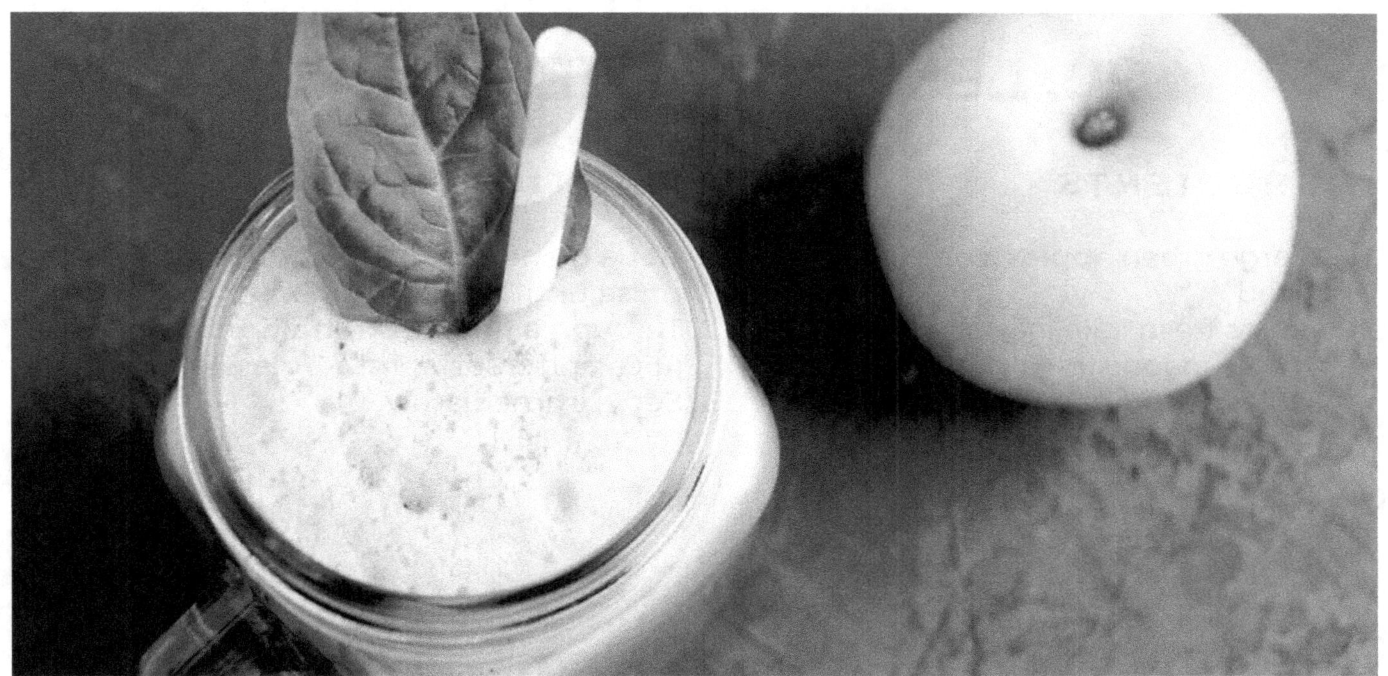

19. APPLE & CUCUMBER JUICE

INGREDIENTS

- 3 large apples, cored and sliced
- 2 large cucumbers, sliced
- 4 celery stalks
- 1 (1-inch) piece fresh ginger, peeled
- 1 lemon, peeled

DIRECTIONS

1. Add all ingredients into a juicer and extract the juice according to the manufacturer's method.
2. Pour into 2 glasses and serve immediately.

Nutritions: *Calories 230, Total Fat 1.1 g, Saturated Fat 0.1 g, Cholesterol 0 mg Sodium 37 mg, Total Carbs 59.5 g, Fiber 10.5 g, Sugar 40.5 g, Protein 3.3 g*

20. LEMONY GREEN JUICE

INGREDIENTS

- 2 large green apples, cored and sliced
- 4 cups fresh kale leaves
- 4 tablespoons fresh parsley leaves
- Tablespoon fresh ginger, peeled
- 1 lemon, peeled
- ½ cup filtered water
- Pinch of salt

DIRECTIONS

1. Get a blender, put all your ingredients and pulse until well combined.
2. Through a fine mesh strainer, strain the juice and transfer into 2 glasses.
3. Serve immediately.

Nutritions: *Calories 196, Total Fat 0.6 g, Saturated Fat 0.1 g, Cholesterol 0mg Sodium 143 mg, Total Carbs 47.9 g, Fiber 8.2 g, Sugar 23.5 g, Protein 5.2 g*

PREPARATION: 10 MIN   **COOKING: 6 MIN**   **SERVES: 2**

21. KALE SCRAMBLE

INGREDIENTS

- 4 eggs
- 1/8 teaspoon ground turmeric
- Salt and ground black pepper, to taste
- 1 tablespoon water
- 2 teaspoons olive oil
- 1 cup fresh kale, tough ribs removed and chopped

DIRECTIONS

1. In a bowl, add the eggs, turmeric, salt, black pepper, and water. With a whisk, beat until foamy.
2. In a wok, heat the oil over medium heat.
3. Add the egg mixture and stir to combine.
4. Immediately, reduce the heat to medium-low and cook for about 1–2 minutes, stirring frequently.
5. Stir in the kale and cook for about 3–4 minutes, just like before.
6. Remove from the heat and serve immediately.

Nutritions: *Calories 183, Total Fat 13.4 g, Saturated Fat 3.4 g, Cholesterol 327mg, Sodium 216 mg, Total Carbs 4.3 g, Fiber 0.5 g, Sugar 0.7 g, Protein 12.1 g*

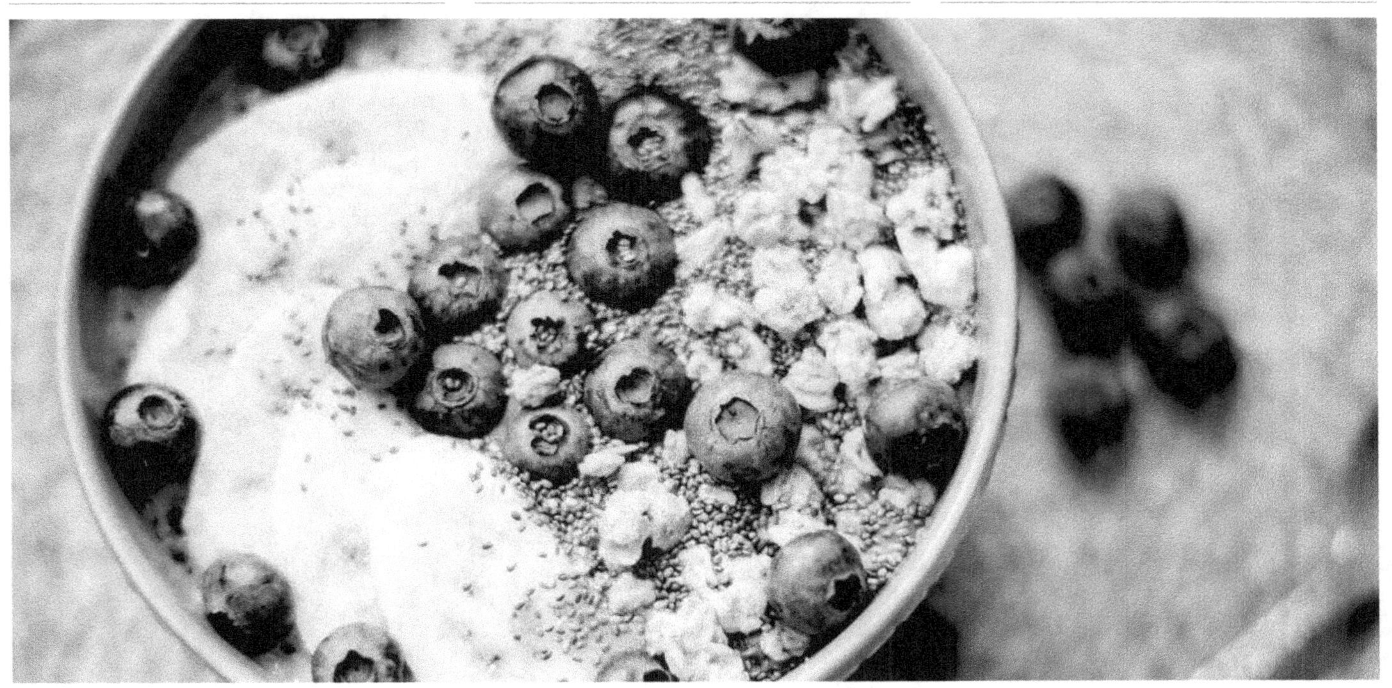

22. BUCKWHEAT PORRIDGE

INGREDIENTS

- 1 cup buckwheat, rinsed
- 1 cup unsweetened almond milk
- 1 cup water
- ½ teaspoon ground cinnamon
- ½ teaspoon vanilla extract
- 1–2 tablespoons raw honey
- ¼ cup fresh blueberries

DIRECTIONS

1. Add all the ingredients in a pan (except honey and blueberries) over medium-high heat and bring to a boil.
2. Now, reduce the heat to low and simmer, covered, for about 10 minutes.
3. Stir in the honey and remove from the heat.
4. Set aside, covered, for about 5 minutes.
5. With a fork, fluff the mixture, and transfer into serving bowls.
6. Top with blueberries and serve.

Nutritions: *Calories 358, Total Fat 4.7 g, Saturated Fat 0.8 g, Cholesterol 0mg, Sodium 95 mg, Total Carbs 3.7 g, Fiber 9.8 g, Sugar 10.6 g, Protein 12 g*

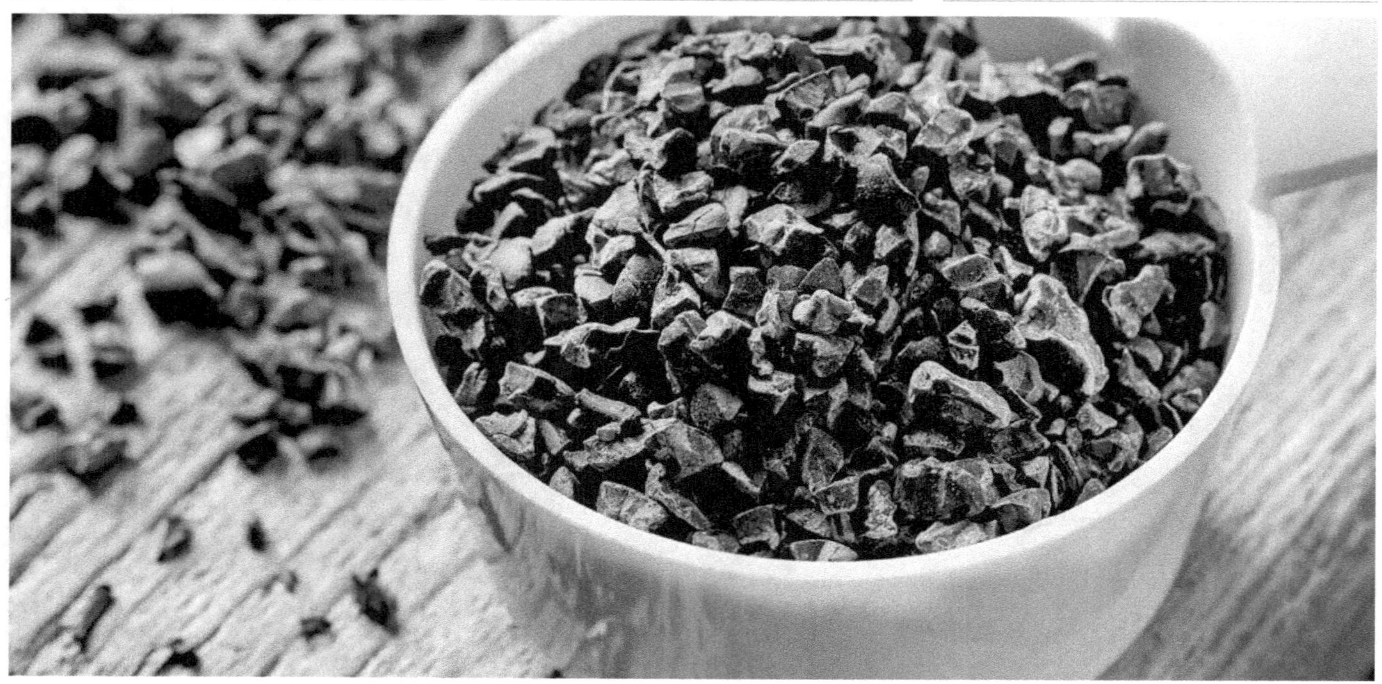

23. CHOCOLATE GRANOLA

INGREDIENTS

- ¼ cup cacao powder
- ¼ cup maple syrup
- 2 tablespoons coconut oil, melted
- ½ teaspoon vanilla extract
- 1/8 teaspoon salt
- 2 cups gluten-free rolled oats
- ¼ cup unsweetened coconut flakes
- 2 tablespoons chia seeds
- 2 tablespoons unsweetened dark chocolate, chopped finely

Nutritions: *Calories 193*
Total Fat 9.1 g, Saturated Fat 5.2 g
Cholesterol 0 mg
Sodium 37 mg, Total Carbs 26.1 g
Fiber 4.6 g, Sugar 5.9 g, Protein 5 g

DIRECTIONS

1. Preheat the oven to 300°F and wrap a medium baking sheet with parchment paper.
2. In a medium pan, add the cacao powder, maple syrup, coconut oil, vanilla extract, and salt, and mix well.
3. Now, place the pan over medium heat and cook for about 2–3 minutes, or until thick and syrupy, stirring continuously.
4. Remove from the heat and set aside.
5. Add the oats, coconut, and chia seeds, in a large bowl and mix well.
6. Add the syrup mixture and mix until well combined.
7. Transfer the granola mixture onto a prepared baking sheet and spread in an even layer.
8. Bake for about 35 minutes.
9. Remove from the oven and set aside for about 1 hour.
10. Add the chocolate pieces and stir to combine.
11. Serve immediately.

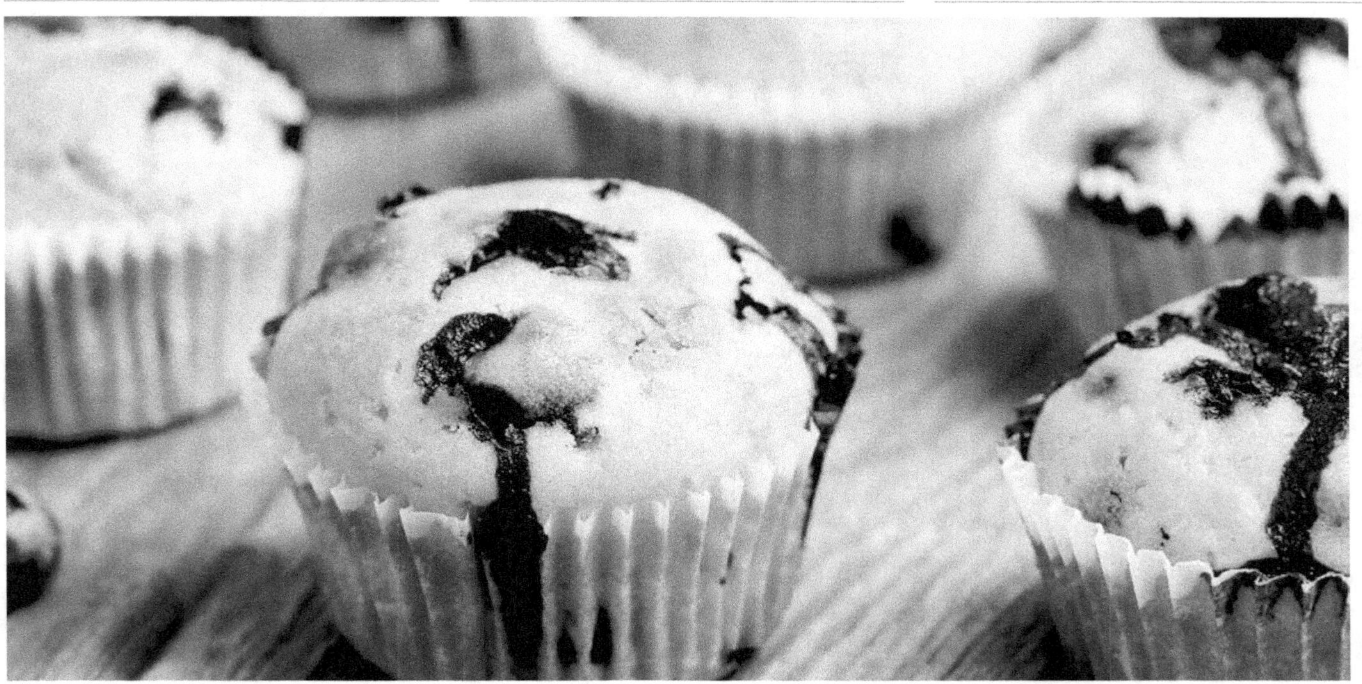

24. BLUEBERRY MUFFINS

INGREDIENTS

- 1 cup buckwheat flour
- ¼ cup arrowroot starch
- 1½ teaspoons baking powder
- ¼ teaspoon sea salt
- 2 eggs
- ½ cup unsweetened almond milk
- 2–3 tablespoons maple syrup
- 2 tablespoons coconut oil, melted
- 1 cup fresh blueberries

Nutritions: *Calories 136, Total Fat 5.3 g, Saturated Fat 3.4 g, Cholesterol 41mg, Sodium 88 mg, Total Carbs 20.7 g, Fiber 2.2 g, Sugar 5.7 g, Protein 3.5 g*

DIRECTIONS

1. Preheat the oven to 350°F and put 8 cups of a muffin tin.
2. In a bowl, place the buckwheat flour, arrowroot starch, baking powder, and salt, and mix well.
3. In a separate bowl, place the eggs, almond milk, maple syrup, and coconut oil, and beat until well combined.
4. Now, place the flour mixture and mix until combined.
5. Gently, fold in the blueberries.
6. Transfer the mixture into prepared muffin cups evenly.
7. Bake for about 25 minutes or until a toothpick inserted in the center comes out clean.
8. Remove the muffin tin from the oven and place it onto a wire rack to cool for about 10 minutes.
9. Carefully invert the muffins onto the wire rack to cool completely before serving.

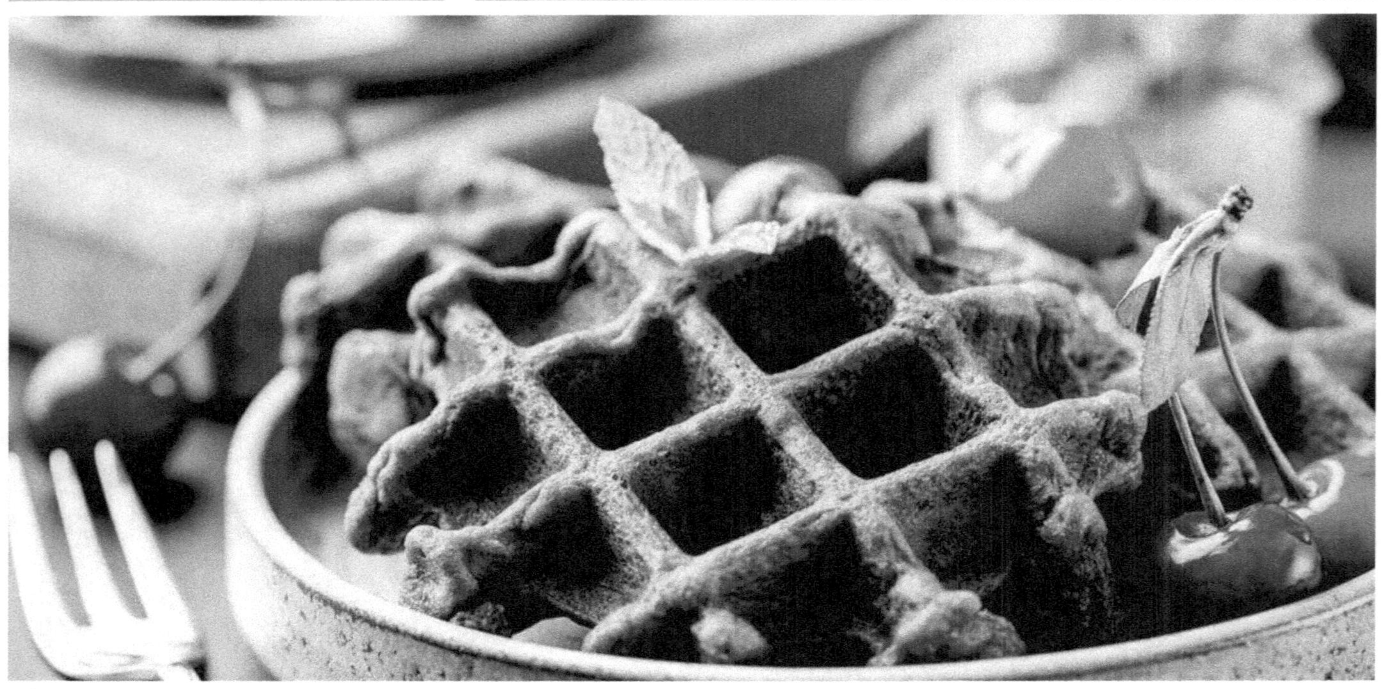

25. CHOCOLATE WAFFLES

INGREDIENTS

- 2 cups unsweetened almond milk
- 1 tablespoon fresh lemon juice
- 1 cup buckwheat flour
- ½ cup cacao powder
- ¼ cup flaxseed meal
- 1 teaspoon baking soda
- 1 teaspoon baking powder
- ¼ teaspoons kosher salt
- 2 large eggs
- ½ cup coconut oil, melted
- ¼ cup dark brown sugar
- 2 teaspoons vanilla extract
- 2 ounces unsweetened dark chocolate, chopped roughly

DIRECTIONS

1. Add the almond milk and lemon juice in a bowl and mix well.
2. Set aside for about 10 minutes.
3. In a bowl, place buckwheat flour, cacao powder, flaxseed meal, baking soda, baking powder, and salt, and mix well.
4. In the bowl of the almond milk mixture, place the eggs, coconut oil, brown sugar, and vanilla extract, and beat until smooth.
5. Now, place the flour mixture and do the same.
6. Gently fold in the chocolate pieces.
7. Preheat the waffle iron and then grease it.
8. Place the desired amount of the mixture into the preheated waffle iron and cook for about 3 minutes, or until golden brown.
9. Repeat with the remaining mixture.

Nutritions: *Calories 295, Total Fat 22.1 g, Saturated Fat 15.5 g, Cholesterol 47mg, Sodium 302 mg, Total Carbs 1.5 g, Fiber 5.2 g, Sugar 5.1 g, Protein 6.3 g*

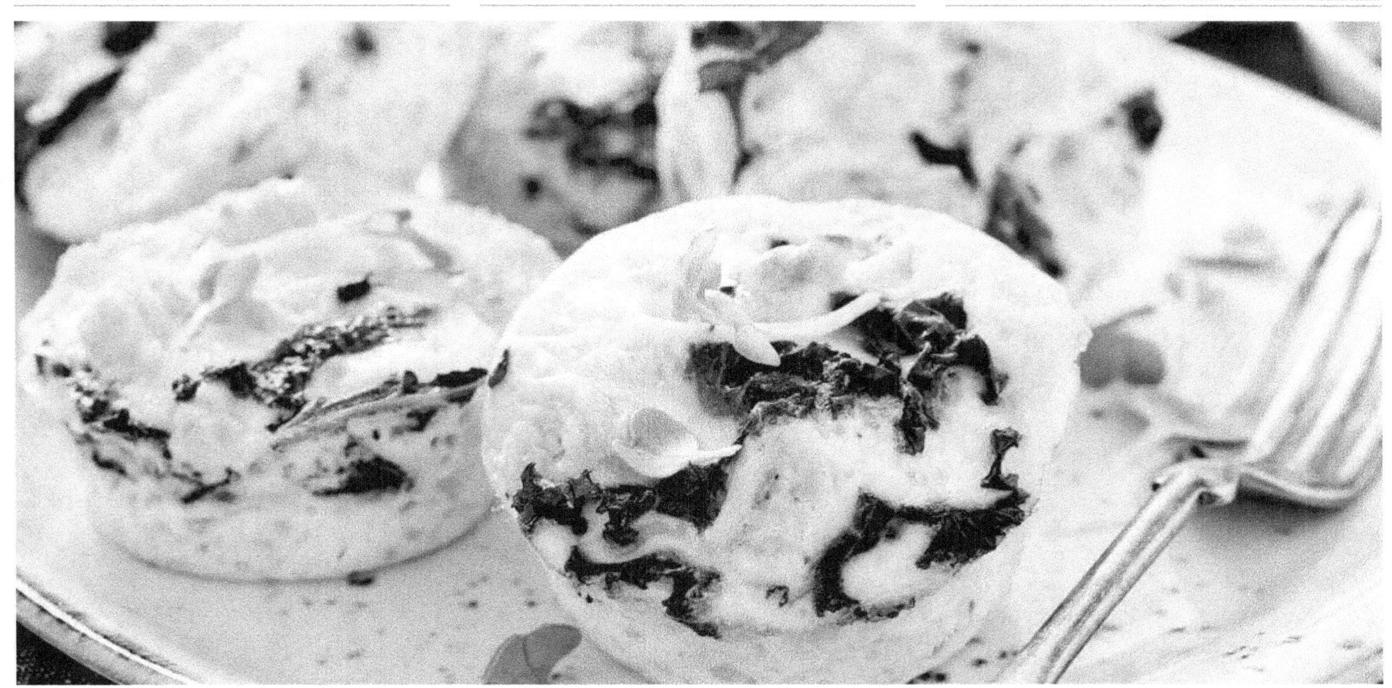

26. SALMON & KALE OMELET

INGREDIENTS

- 6 eggs
- 2 tablespoons unsweetened almond milk
- Salt and ground black pepper, to taste
- 2 tablespoons olive oil
- 4 ounces smoked salmon, cut into bite-sized chunks
- 2 cup fresh kale, tough ribs removed and chopped finely
- 4 scallions, chopped finely

DIRECTIONS

1. In a bowl, place the eggs, coconut milk, salt, and black pepper, and beat well. Set aside.
2. In a non-stick wok, heat the oil over medium heat.
3. Place the egg mixture evenly and cook for about 30 seconds without stirring.
4. Place the salmon kale and scallions on top of the egg mixture evenly.
5. Now, reduce heat to low.
6. With the lid, cover the wok and cook for about 4–5 minutes or until the omelet is done completely.
7. Uncover the wok and cook for about 1 minute.
8. Carefully transfer the omelet onto a serving plate and serve.

Nutritions: *Calories 210, Total Fat 14.9 g, Saturated Fat 3.3 g, Cholesterol252mg, Sodium 682 mg, Total Carbs 5.2 g, Fiber 0.9 g, Sugar 0.9 g, Protein 14.8 g*

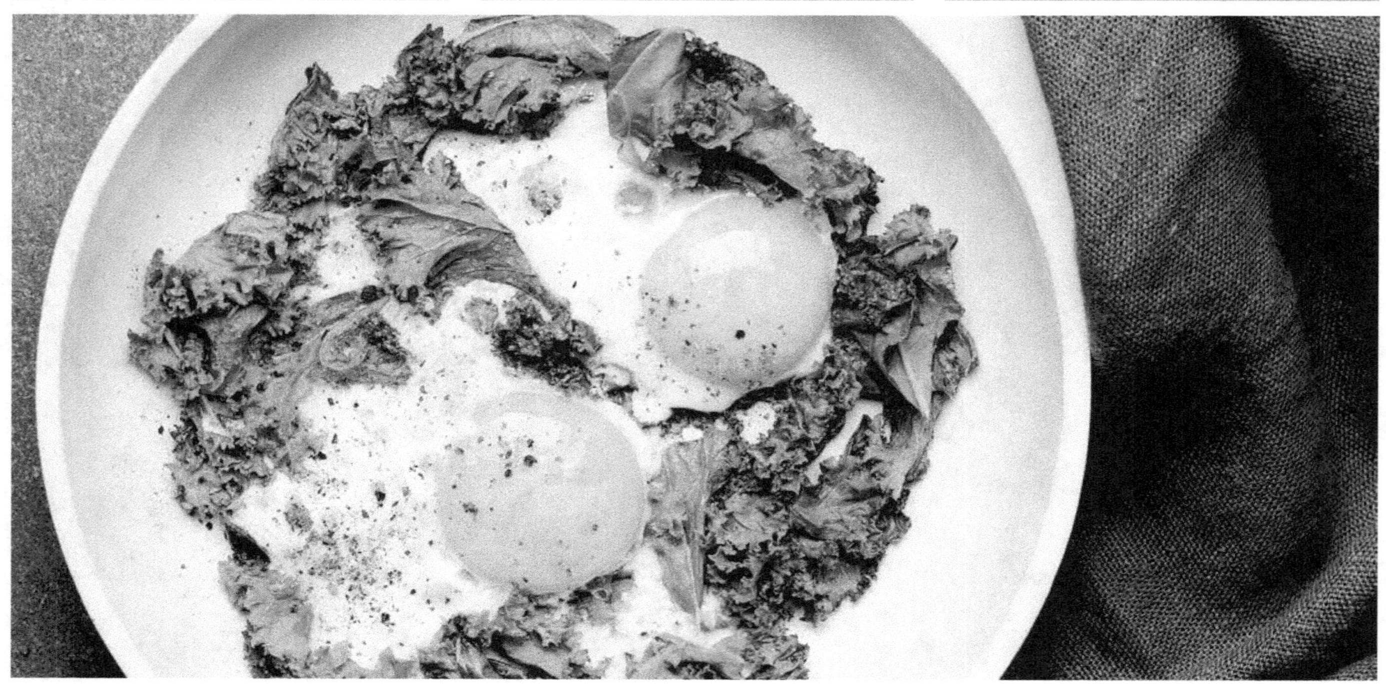

27. EGGS WITH KALE

INGREDIENTS

- 2 tablespoons olive oil
- 1 yellow onion, chopped
- 2 garlic cloves, minced
- 1 cup tomatoes, chopped
- ½ pound fresh kale, tough ribs removed and chopped
- 1 teaspoon ground cumin
- ¼ teaspoon red pepper flakes, crushed
- Salt and ground black pepper, to taste
- 4 eggs
- 2 tablespoons fresh parsley, chopped

DIRECTIONS

1. Heat the oil in a large wok over medium heat and sauté the onion for about 4–5 minutes.
2. Add garlic and sauté for about 1 minute.
3. Add the tomatoes, spices, salt, and black pepper. Cook for about 2–3 minutes, stirring frequently.
4. Stir in the kale and cook for about 4–5 minutes.
5. Carefully crack eggs on top of the kale mixture.
6. With the lid, cover the wok and cook for about 10 minutes, or until desired doneness of the eggs.
7. Serve hot with the garnishing of parsley.

Nutritions: *Calories 175, Total Fat 11.7 g, Saturated Fat 2.4 g, Cholesterol 164 mg Sodium 130 mg, Total Carbs 11.5 g, Fiber 2.2 g, Sugar 2.8 g, Protein 8.2 g*

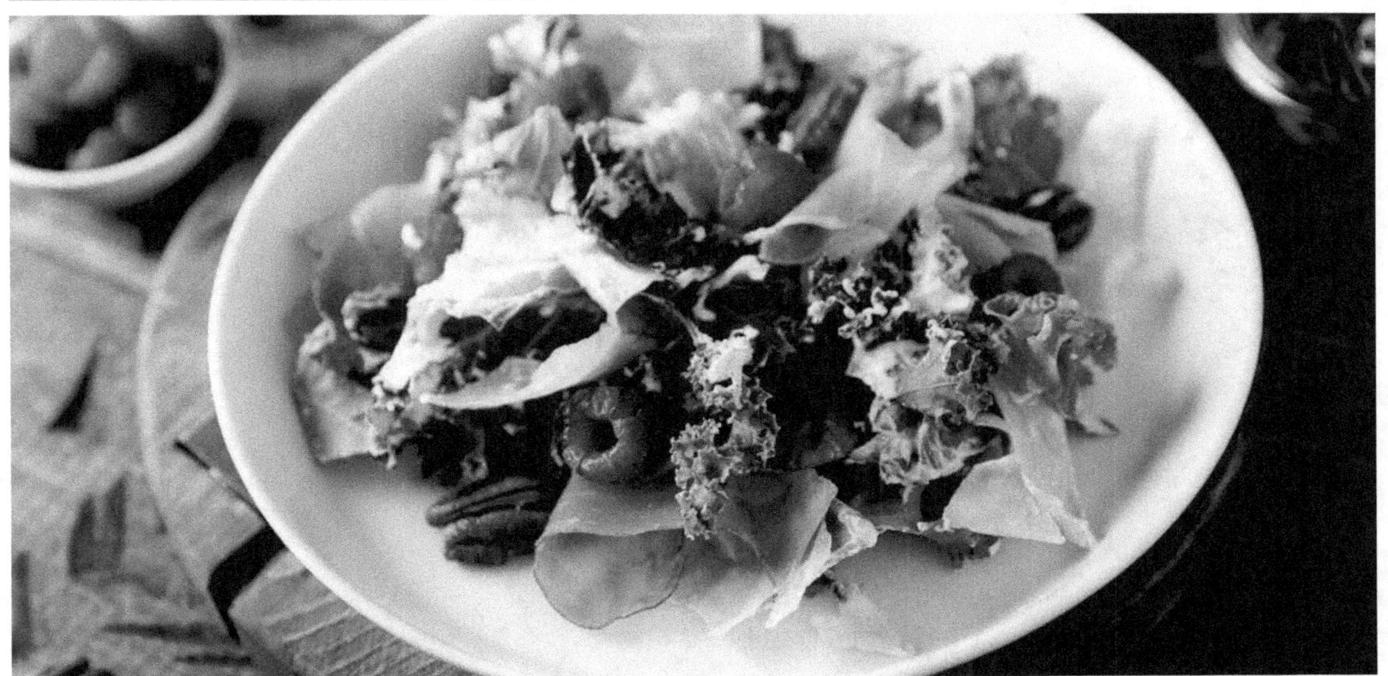

28. KALE & RASPBERRY SALAD

INGREDIENTS

- 3 cups fresh baby kale
- ½ cup fresh raspberries
- ¼ cup walnuts, chopped

Dressing:

- 1 tablespoon extra-virgin olive oil
- 1 tablespoon apple cider vinegar
- ½ teaspoon pure maple syrup
- Salt and ground black pepper, to taste

DIRECTIONS

For salad:

1. In a salad bowl, place all ingredients and mix.

For dressing:

1. Place all ingredients in another bowl and beat until well combined.
2. Place dressing on top of the salad and toss to coat well.
3. Serve immediately.

Nutritions: *Calories 228, Total Fat 16.4 g, Saturated Fat 1.5 g, Cholesterol 0 mg Sodium 122 mg, Total Carbs 16.9 g, Fiber 4.6 g, Sugar 2.6 g, Protein 7.1 g*

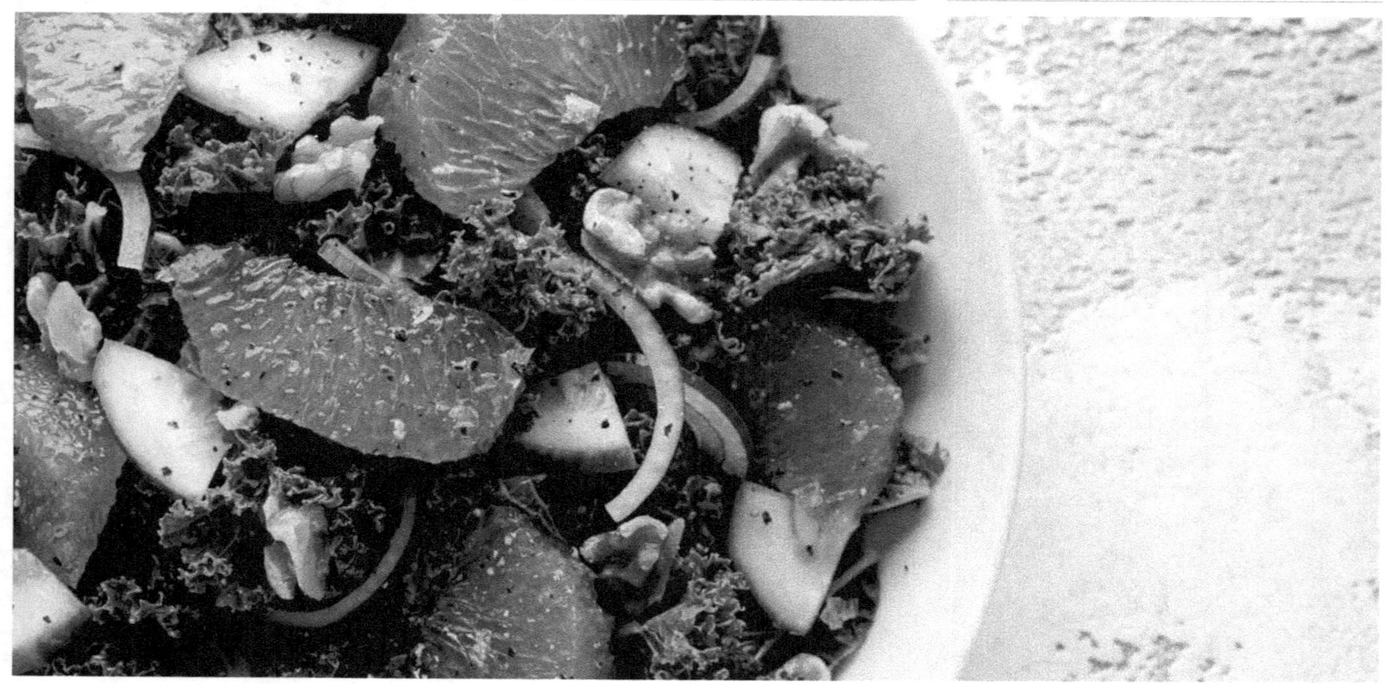

29. KALE & CITRUS FRUIT SALAD

INGREDIENTS

Salad:

- 3 cups fresh kale, tough ribs removed and torn
- 1 orange, peeled and segmented
- 1 grapefruit, peeled and segmented
- 2 tablespoons unsweetened dried cranberries
- ¼ teaspoon white sesame seeds

Dressing:

- 2 tablespoons extra-virgin olive oil
- 2 tablespoons fresh orange juice
- 1 teaspoon Dijon mustard
- ½ teaspoon raw honey
- Salt and ground black pepper, to taste

DIRECTIONS

For salad:

1. In a salad bowl, place all ingredients and mix.

For dressing:

1. Place all ingredients in another bowl and beat until well combined.
2. Place dressing on top of the salad and toss to coat well.
3. Serve immediately.

Nutritions: *Calories 256, Total Fat 14.5g, Saturated Fat 2.1 g, Cholesterol 0 mg Sodium 150 mg, Total Carbs 31.3 g, Fiber 4.8 g, Sugar 16.6 g, Protein 4.6 g*

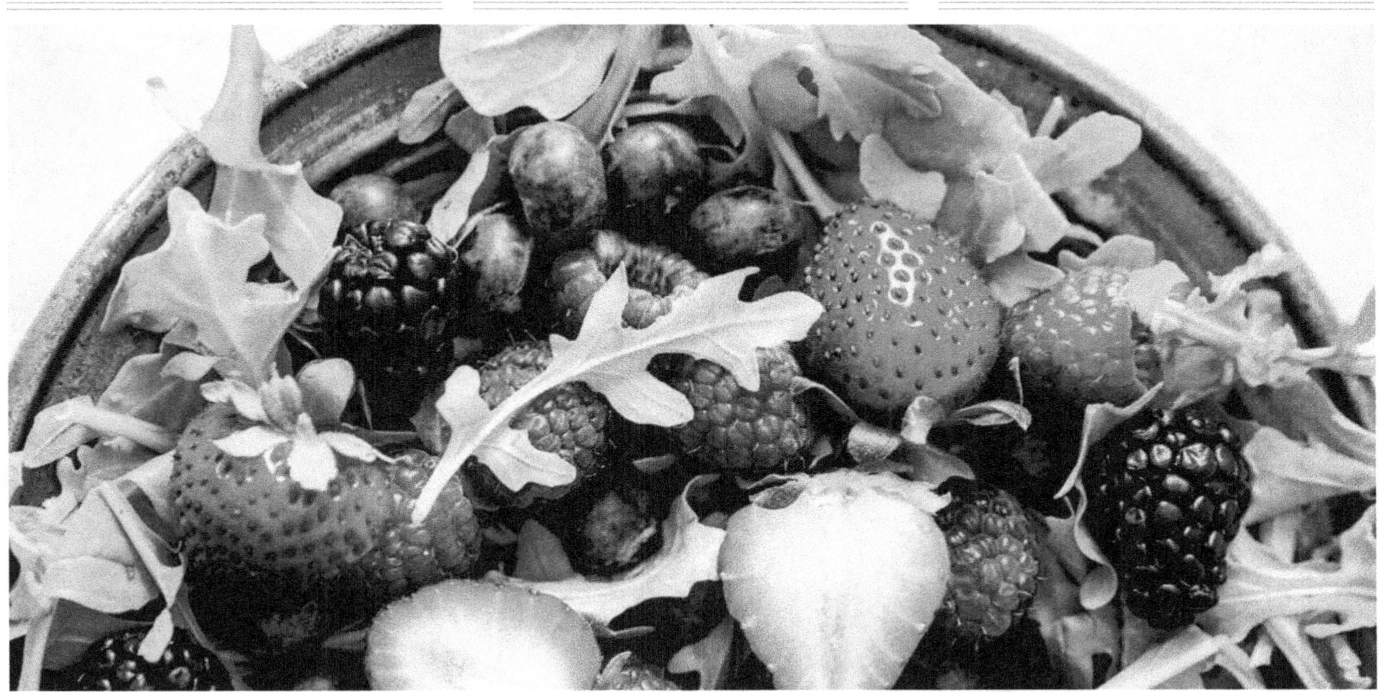

30. ARUGULA & BERRIES SALAD

INGREDIENTS

- 1 cup fresh strawberries, hulled and sliced
- ½ cup fresh blackberries
- ½ cup fresh blueberries
- ½ cup fresh raspberries
- 6 cups fresh arugula
- 2 tablespoons extra-virgin olive oil
- Salt and ground black pepper, to taste

DIRECTIONS

1. In a salad bowl, place all the ingredients and toss to coat well.
2. Serve immediately.

Nutritions: *Calories 105, Total Fat 7.6 g, Saturated Fat 1 g, Cholesterol 0 mg Sodium 48 mg, Total Carbs 10.1 g, Fiber 3.6 g, Sugar 5.7 g, Protein 1.6 g*

LUNCH RECIPES

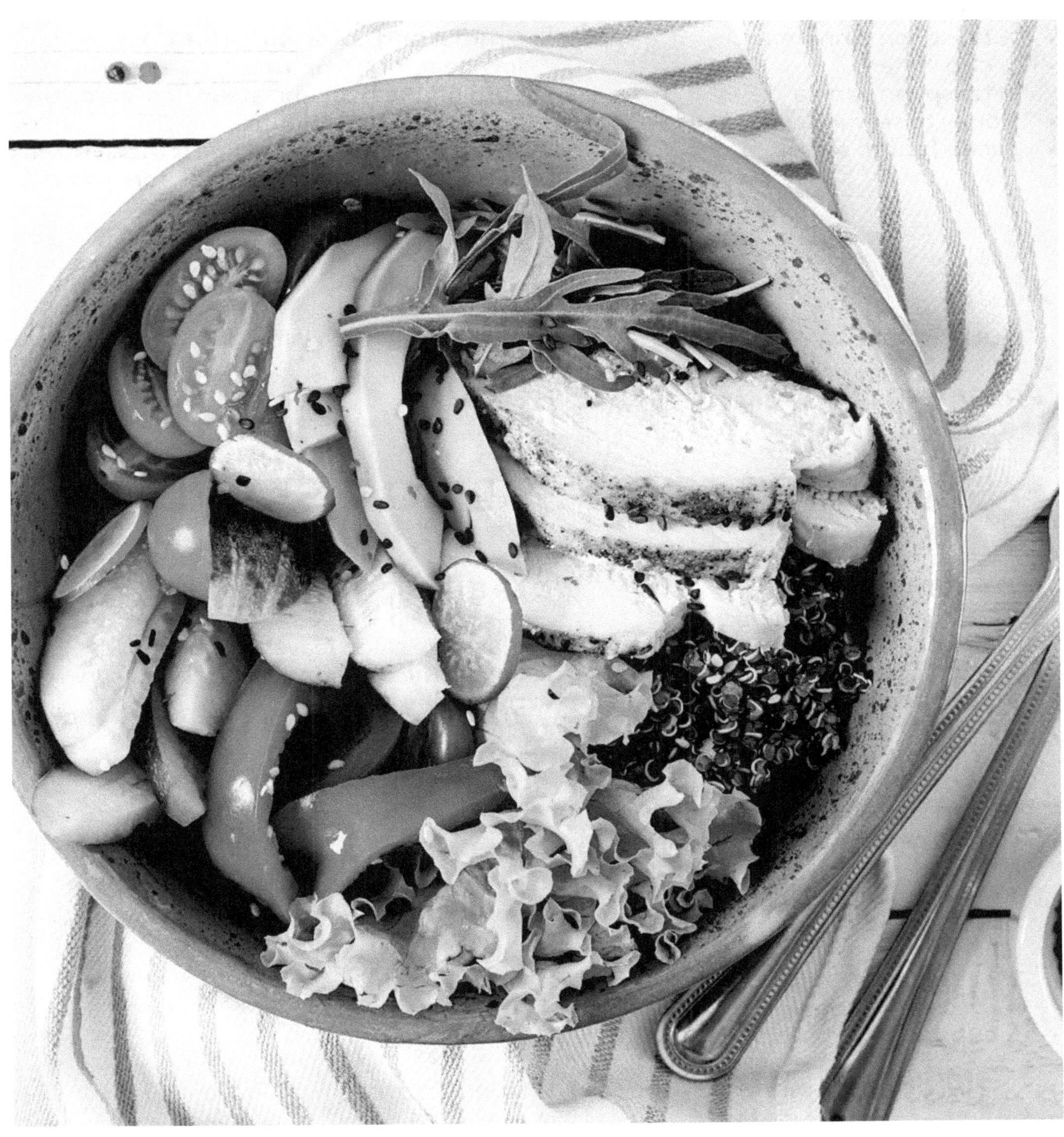

31. CINNAMON BUCKWHEAT BOWLS

INGREDIENTS

- ½ cup buckwheat groats, rinsed
- ½ cup almond milk or milk of choice
- ½ teaspoon cinnamon
- ½ cup water
- ½ teaspoon vanilla
- Honey to serve
- Sliced fruit to serve

DIRECTIONS

1. In a small saucepan, add washed buckwheat grains, water, almond milk, cinnamon, and vanilla. Boil and then simmer and cover with a lid. Cook over low heat for 10 minutes.
2. Turn off the heat and steam, covered, for an additional 5 minutes.
3. Pour with a fork and divide it into a bowl. Fill with fruit slices, sprinkle more milk and chopped honey if desired.

Nutritions: *Calories 182, Fat 1 g, Carbohydrates 34 g, Protein 6.7 g*

32. SIRTFOOD SALMON SALAD

INGREDIENTS

- 1 cup rocket
- 2 oz. chicory leaves
- 1 tablespoon capers
- 3 oz. avocado, peeled, stoned and sliced
- 3.5 oz. smoked salmon slices
- 1/8 cup walnuts, chopped
- 1 large medjool date, pitted and chopped
- Juice of ¼ lemon
- 1 tablespoon extra-virgin olive oil
- 3/8 cup parsley, chopped
- ½ oz. celery leaves
- ¼ cup red onion, sliced

DIRECTIONS

1. Place the salad leaves in a big bowl.
2. Mix all the other ingredients and serve on the leaves.

Nutritions: *Calories 194, Fat 9 g, Carbohydrates 4.5 g, Protein 21 g*

33. ARUGULA, EGG, AND CHARRED ASPARAGUS SALAD

INGREDIENTS

- 12 oz. medium asparagus, trimmed
- ½ teaspoon black pepper, divided
- 4 large eggs in shells
- 1 tablespoon fresh lemon juice
- 5 oz. baby arugula
- 1 tablespoon extra-virgin olive oil
- 1 tablespoon water
- ¼ cup plain whole-milk Greek yogurt
- 1 teaspoon kosher salt, divided

DIRECTIONS

1. Preheat broiler to high.
2. Bring a small saucepan filled with water to a boil. Carefully add eggs. Cook for 8 minutes. Place eggs in a bowl filled with ice water and let stand for 2 minutes. Peel eggs, cut into quarters and sprinkle with ¼ teaspoon salt and 1/8 teaspoon pepper.
3. Combine olive oil, ¼ teaspoon salt, ¼ teaspoon pepper, and asparagus on a baking sheet. Spread in a single layer in pan. Boil for 3 minutes or until lightly charred. Remove asparagus mixture from the pan and cut into 2 inch pieces.
4. Combine remaining ¼ teaspoon salt, remaining 1/8 teaspoon pepper, yogurt, juice, and 1 tablespoon water in a medium bowl, stirring with a whisk. Add arugula and toss. Arrange arugula mixture on a platter. Top with asparagus mixture and eggs. Enjoy!

Nutritions: *Calories 147, Fat 9.1 g, Carbohydrates 6 g, Protein 10 g*

34. SPRING VEGETABLE AND QUINOA SALAD WITH BACON

INGREDIENTS

- 1 ¾ cups ginger-coconut quinoa
- 2.5 cups fresh asparagus, cut diagonally into 1 inch pieces
- 3 center-cut bacon slices, chopped
- 1 tablespoon unsalted butter
- 3 tablespoons cider vinegar
- ½ cup frozen green peas
- 2 teaspoons whole-grain Dijon mustard
- 5 oz. baby spinach
- 3 tablespoons sliced almonds, toasted
- 1 teaspoon black pepper
- 1 tablespoon fresh thyme leaves
- 1 tablespoon chopped fresh tarragon
- ½ cup chopped fresh flat-leaf parsley

DIRECTIONS

1. Boil a large pot filled with water. Add asparagus and peas. Boil for 2 minutes, then drain. Plunge into a bowl of ice water and drain.
2. Cook the bacon in a large saucepan over medium-high heat, stirring occasionally. Remove bacon from the pan with a slotted spoon. Set aside.
3. Add vinegar, butter, and Dijon mustard to drippings in the pan, stirring with a whisk until butter melts. Add quinoa and pepper to the pan—cook for 1 minute.
4. Place quinoa mixture in a medium bowl. Add asparagus mixture, parsley, tarragon, thyme, and spinach, tossing to combine. Divide quinoa mixture among 4 plates; sprinkle evenly with reserved bacon and almonds.

Nutritions: *Calories 263, Fat 9.8 g, Carbohydrates 28 g, Protein 7 g*

35. GOLDEN CHICORY IN PROSCIUTTO WRAPS

INGREDIENTS

- 2 heads of chicory
- 4 slices prosciutto or Serrano ham
- 75 ml vegetable stock or white wine
- 2 tablespoons butter
- 2 tablespoons Dijon mustard
- ¼ cup whipping cream
- 2 thyme sprigs
- 4 slices, about 2 oz. melting cheese (cheddar is great)
- Sauté potatoes and green salad to serve

DIRECTIONS

1. Preheat oven to 350 °F. Cut a cross from the base in the middle of the end of each chicory head. Fill the butter in the grooves, and then place the slices of Serrano ham in pairs on the work surface, overlapping them slightly. Paint the ham with mustard and spread the radish on top. Pull each radish head away from you, comfortably wrapping it in the ham.
2. Place the radish wrapped in an oven or small skillet, pour over the vegetable stock or white wine on top with the thyme sprigs. Cover the plate with loose foil and bake for 30-40 minutes until the radish is soft.
3. Unlock the plate, place the cheese slices on the chicory and bake, keep uncovered for another 6-8 minutes, until the cheese is melted and browned. The radish is now ready to serve. For an extra touch, remove the chicory, place the pan on medium heat and boil the juices with the cream for 4-5 minutes until they are rich and syrupy.
4. Pour the sauce over the radish. Serve with sautéed potatoes and salad.

Nutritions: *Calories 493, Fat 36 g, Carbohydrates 9 g, Protein 32 g*

36. VEGETABLE CABBAGE SOUP

INGREDIENTS

- ½ large head cabbage, chopped
- 1 large onion, chopped
- 2 stalks celery, minced
- 2 carrots, chopped
- 2 tablespoons extra virgin olive oil
- 2 cloves garlic, minced
- ½ teaspoon chili powder
- 1 can white beans, drained and rinsed
- 1 can chopped fire-roasted tomatoes
- 1 pinch red pepper flakes
- 1 teaspoon thyme leaves
- 4 cups low-sodium vegetable broth
- 2 tablespoons freshly of chopped parsley, and more for garnish
- Kosher salt
- Freshly ground black pepper
- 2 cups water

DIRECTIONS

1. In a large pot over medium heat, heat olive oil. Add onion, celery, and carrots, and season with salt, pepper, and chili powder. Cook, stirring often, until vegetables are soft, 5 to 6 minutes. Stir in beans, thyme, and garlic and cook until garlic is fragrant, about 30 seconds. Add broth and water, and bring to a simmer.
2. Stir in tomatoes and cabbage and simmer until cabbage is wilted, about 6 minutes.
3. Remove from heat and stir in red pepper flakes, and parsley. Season to taste with salt and pepper. Garnish with more parsley, if desired. Enjoy!

Nutritions: *Calories 92, Fat 0.8 g, Carbohydrates 11.6 g, Protein 2.5 g*

37. FRESH HERB FRITTATA

INGREDIENTS

- 8 fresh eggs
- 3 tablespoons chopped fresh parsley
- 2 tablespoons chopped fresh oregano
- 4 scallions, sliced thin, using both white and green parts
- ½ cup heavy cream
- ¾ cup finely grated parmesan cheese, divided into ½ cup and 1/4 cup portions
- Salt and pepper to taste

DIRECTIONS

1. Preheat oven to 400 ˚F.
2. In a medium mixing bowl, combine eggs, parsley, scallions, oregano, ½ cup of cheese, and heavy cream. Whisk together until thoroughly combined—season with salt and pepper, to taste.
3. In a 10-inch spicy cast iron pot, heat about 1 tablespoon of olive oil over medium heat.
4. Add the egg mixture and cook for about 5 minutes or until the edges start to come out.
5. Sprinkle the remaining cup of cheese over the eggs.
6. Transfer the skillet to the oven and bake for 10-12 minutes, or until the fritters are puffy, the edges are visible and shake a little in the center.
7. Bake on low for about 30-45 seconds to brown the lid.

Nutritions: *Calories 105, Fat 2.8 g, Carbohydrates 5 g*

38. HERB-ROASTED OLIVES AND TOMATOES

INGREDIENTS

- 1 cup Greek olives
- 1 cup garlic-stuffed olives
- 2 cups cherry tomatoes
- 1 cup pitted ripe olives
- 1 tablespoon herbs de Provence
- 3 tablespoons olive oil
- 8 garlic cloves, peeled
- ¼ teaspoon pepper

DIRECTIONS

1. Preheat oven to 425 °F.
2. Combine cherry tomatoes, garlic-stuffed olives, Greek olives, pitted ripe olives, and garlic cloves on a greased baking pan. Add oil and seasonings. Toss to coat. Roast until tomatoes are softened, 15-20 minutes, stirring occasionally.

Nutritions: *Calories 69, Fat 6 g, Carbohydrates 3 g, Protein 0.5 g*

39. GRILLED ASPARAGUS WITH CAPER VINAIGRETTE

INGREDIENTS

- 1 ½ pounds asparagus spears, trimmed
- 2 teaspoons caper, coarsely chopped
- 1 tablespoon red wine vinegar
- 1 garlic clove, minced
- 3 tablespoons extra virgin olive oil
- ¼ cup small basil leaves
- ½ teaspoon Dijon mustard
- Cooking spray
- ½ teaspoon kosher salt, divided
- ¼ teaspoon freshly ground black pepper

DIRECTIONS

1. Preheat grill to medium-high heat.
2. Place asparagus in a shallow dish. Add 1 tablespoon oil and ¼ teaspoon salt, tossing well to coat. Place asparagus on grill rack coated with cooking spray. Grill 4 minutes or until crisp-tender, turning after 2 minutes.
3. Combine remaining ¼ teaspoon salt, vinegar, mustard, and garlic. Stir with a whisk. Slowly pour remaining 2 tablespoons oil into vinegar mixture, stirring constantly with a whisk. Stir in capers. Arrange asparagus on a serving platter. Drizzle with vinaigrette, and sprinkle with basil.

Nutritions: *Calories 89, Fat 6.9 g, Carbohydrates 4.7 g, Protein 2.8 g*

40. HERBY PORK WITH APPLE & CHICORY SALAD

INGREDIENTS

- 14 oz. pork tenderloin, trimmed of any sinew and fat
- 2 large apples, cored and sliced
- 270g pack chicory, leaves separated
- 1 tablespoon honey
- 1 tablespoon walnut oil
- 1 tablespoon chopped parsley
- 1 tablespoon chopped tarragon
- 2 teaspoons wholegrain mustard
- Juice of 1 lemon

DIRECTIONS

1. Preheat oven to 350°F. Grate pork with 1 teaspoon oil, 1 teaspoon mustard, and a few spices. Brown, transfer to a baking sheet and squeeze half of the herbs. Bake for 15 minutes until well cooked.
2. To make the salad, mix the lemon juice, honey, and the rest of the walnut oil and mustard. Period and add apples, radishes, and other herbs. Serve the sliced pork with the salad on the side.

Nutritions: *Calories 252, Fat 8 g, Carbohydrates 16 g, Protein 22 g*

41. CHIA, QUINOA & AVOCADO SALAD

INGREDIENTS

- ½ cup quinoa
- ¼ cup black chia seeds
- 1 avocado
- ¾ cup feta cheese
- 1 red onion
- 1 chili
- 2 tablespoons olive oil
- 1 garlic clove, minced
- 1/8 cup sunflower seeds
- 1 tablespoon agave syrup
- 2 limes
- ½ cup cherry tomatoes
- 1 cup rocket
- Sea salt
- Freshly ground pepper

DIRECTIONS

1. Pour the quinoa into a sieve and rinse with cold water for a few minutes to rinse off the soap. Tip in a saucepan. Pour in 1 cup of boiling water. Cover and boil. Lower the heat and simmer for 10-12 minutes until the water is absorbed and the quinoa is smooth. Take out from the fire.
2. While the quinoa is simmering, pour the chia seeds into a dry skillet. Toast over medium heat for 3-4 minutes until the chia seeds smell fragrant—tip in a large bowl. Add the sunflower seeds to the pan and toast for 2 minutes. Add the chia seeds to the bowl. Mix the quinoa in the bowl.
3. Peel a pumpkin, grate it and chop the onion. Add them with the cherry tomatoes to the bowl—half and half avocado. Remove the stone and remove the meat from the skin. Chop it and add it to the bowl. Finely chop the leaves of the rocket and add them to the bowl. Throw it all together.
4. Pour the limes into a small bowl. Add olive oil and agave syrup—half chili. Remove the seeds and white pieces for less heat and chop the chili. Peel a pumpkin, grate it and squeeze the garlic. Add to the lime juice with a pinch of salt and pepper. Lightly beat the dressing.
5. Add the sauce to the bowl. Fly to mix. Serve the salad on plates and crumble the feta cheese to serve.

Nutritions: *Calories 212, Fat 11 g, Carbohydrates 29 g, Protein 8 g*

42. TOMATO GREEN BEAN SOUP

INGREDIENTS

- 1 ½ cups diced fresh tomatoes
- ½ cup chopped onion
- ½ pound fresh green beans cut into 1 inch pieces
- ½ cup chopped carrots
- 1/8 cup minced fresh basil
- ½ garlic clove, minced
- ¼ teaspoon salt
- 1/8 teaspoon pepper
- 1 teaspoon butter
- 3 cups reduced-sodium vegetable broth

DIRECTIONS

1. In a large saucepan, sauté onion and carrots in butter for 5 minutes. Stir in the broth, green beans and garlic. Bring to a boil. Reduce heat. Cover and simmer until vegetables are tender.
2. Stir in the tomatoes, basil, salt and pepper. Cover and simmer 5 minutes longer.

Nutritions: *Calories 57, Fat 1.3 g, Carbohydrates 10 g, Protein 5 g*

43. KALE SALAD WITH PECORINO AND LEMON

INGREDIENTS

- 1 large bunch kale, washed and trimmed of steams
- 2 lemons, juiced
- 4 ounces Pecorino Romano, grated
- ½ cup olive oil
- Kosher salt and fresh black pepper to taste

DIRECTIONS

1. Wrap several cabbage leaves lengthwise and, using the tip of a knife, cut off the thick central stem. On the other hand, wrap the remaining pile of dehydrated leaves in a tight cigar shape and cut them into thin ribbons.
2. Discard the grated cabbage with the cheese. Lightly beat the lemon juice and olive oil and pour over the salad. Try and season with salt and pepper. Let the salad sit at room temperature for an hour before serving.

Nutritions: *Calories 238, Fat 15 g, Carbohydrates 21 g, Protein 8 g*

DINNER RECIPES

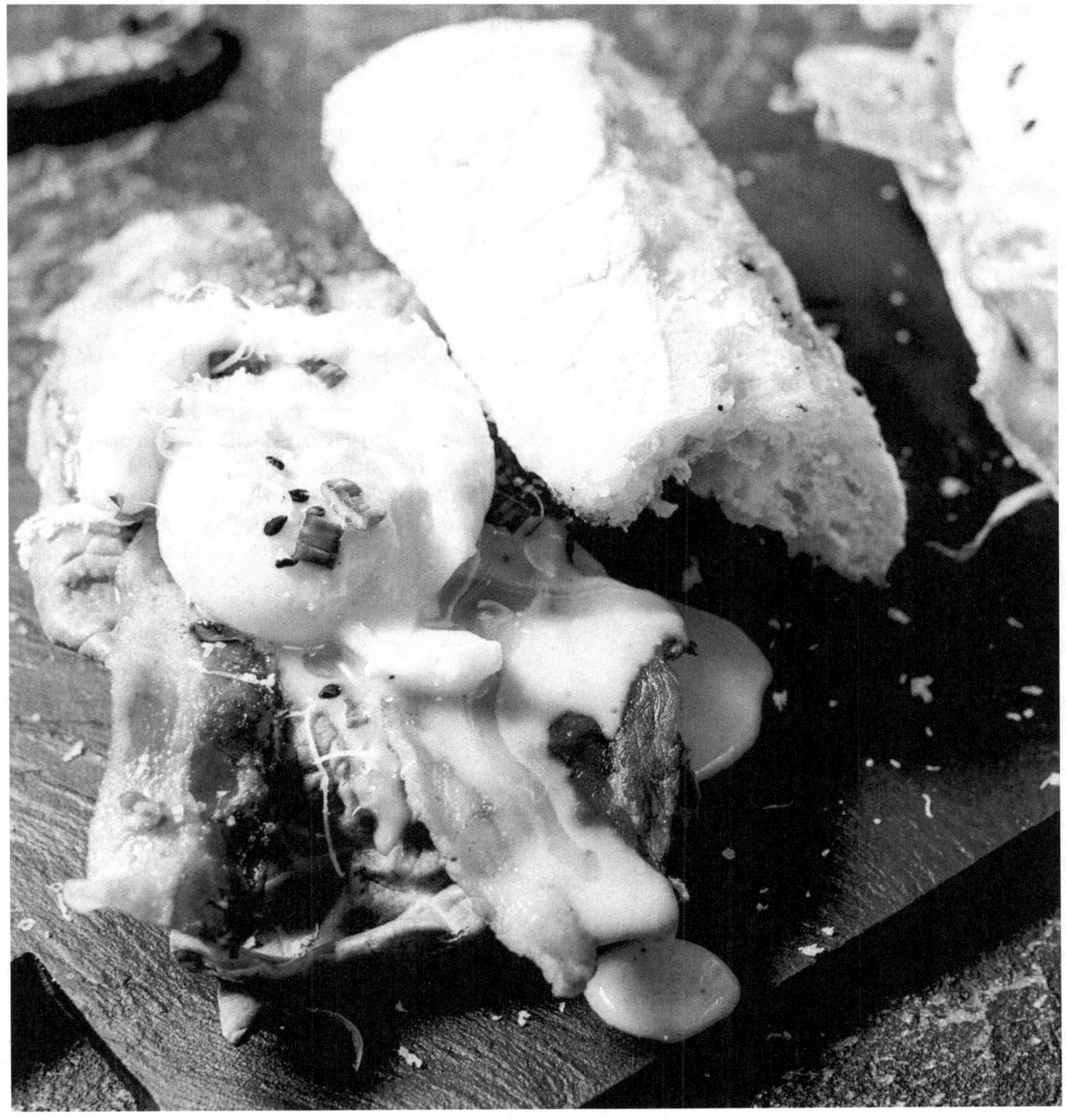

44. BANG-BANG CHICKEN NOODLE STIR-FRY

INGREDIENTS

- 1 tablespoon sunflower oil
- 750g package chicken thighs, boned, any surplus skin trimmed
- 250g frozen chopped mixed peppers
- Inch courgette, peeled into ribbons, seeded center chopped
- 1 chicken stock cube
- 250g pack moderate egg yolks
- 4 garlic cloves, finely chopped
- 1/2 teaspoon crushed chilies, and additional to serve (optional)
- 4 tablespoons reduced-salt soy sauce
- 2 teaspoons caster sugar
- 1 lime, zested, 1/2 juiced, 1/2 slice into wedges to function

DIRECTIONS

1. Heat the oil in a skillet on a medium-low warmth. Fry the chicken skin-side down to 10 minutes or until your skin is emptied. Flip and simmer for 10 minutes, or until cooked. Transfer to a plate cover loosely with foil.
2. Reheat the wok over a high temperature, add the peppers and sliced courgette; simmer for 5 minutes. Meanwhile, bring a bowl of water to the boil, and then crumble in the stock block, adding the noodles. Simmer for 45 minutes until cooked, and then drain well.
3. Insert the garlic and crushed chilies into the wok; simmer for two minutes. In a bowl, mix the soy, sugar and the lime juice and zest. Enhance the wok, bubble for 2 minutes; you can add the courgette noodles and ribbons. Toss with tongs to coat in the sauce.
4. Cut the chicken into pieces. Divide the noodles between 4 bowls and top with the chicken. Serve with the lime wedges along with extra crushed chilies, in case you prefer.

Nutritions: *Power 2995 kj (718 kcal)(36%), Fat 36 g (51%),Saturates 12 g (60%) Sugars 8 g (8%), Salt 2.4 g (39% of those reference ingested), Carbohydrate 55 g Protein 41.3 g, Fiber 5.7 g*

45. CAJUN STEAK AND VEG RICE JAR RECIPE

INGREDIENTS

- 1 tablespoon vegetable oil
- 1 celery stick, finely chopped
- 3 large carrots, sliced into rounds
- 250g frozen chopped mixed peppers
- 4 spring onions, chopped, green and white parts split
- 500g 5% beef mince
- 2 teaspoon seasoning
- 1 teaspoon tomato purée
- 2 x 250g packs ready-cooked long-grain rice

DIRECTIONS

1. Heat the oil in a large, shallow skillet over moderate heat. Add the carrots, celery, peppers, and snowy areas of the nuts. Cook for 10 minutes before the vegetables begin to soften.
2. Insert the mince, season liberally, and cook for 10 minutes before mince is browned and start to really go crispy.
3. Insert the Cajun seasoning and tomato purée; stir fry to coat the mince. Hint inside the rice combined with 4 tablespoons of plain water. Stir to completely unite heat and heat until the rice is hot. Scatter on the rest of the spring onion before serving.

Nutritions: *Power 1925 kj (456 kcal) (23%), Fat 12 g (18%), Saturates 3 g (17%) Sugar 13 g (14%), Salt 1 g (17% of those reference ingested), Carbohydrate 53.1 g Protein 32.8 g, Fiber 8.3 g*

46. PESTO SALMON PASTA NOODLES RECIPE

INGREDIENTS

- 350g penne
- 2 x 212g tins cherry salmon, drained
- 1 lemon, zested and juiced
- 190g jar green pesto
- 250g package cherry tomatoes halved
- 100g bunch spring onions, finely chopped
- 125g package reduced-fat mozzarella

DIRECTIONS

1. Preheat the oven to 220°C, buff 200°C. Boil the pasta for 5 minutes. Drain, reserving 100ml drinking water.
2. Meanwhile, at a 2ltr ovenproof dish, mix the salmon, lemon zest, and juice, then pesto (booking 2 tablespoons) berries and half of the spring onions; season.
3. Mix the pasta and reserved cooking water to the dish. Mix the allowed pesto using 1 tablespoon water and then drizzle on the pasta. Gently within the mozzarella, top with the rest of the spring onions and bake for 25 minutes until golden.

Nutritions: *Power 2815 kj (669 kcal) (33%), Fat 25 g (35%), Saturates 6 g (28%) Sugars 7 g (7%)*

47. SRI LANKAN-STYLE SWEET POTATO CURRY RECIPE

INGREDIENTS

- 1/2 onion, roughly sliced
- 3 garlic cloves, roughly sliced
- 25g sliced ginger, chopped and peeled
- 15g fresh coriander stalks and leaves split leaves sliced
- 2 1/2 tablespoon moderate tikka curry powder
- 60g package cashew nuts
- 1 tablespoon olive oil
- 500g Red Mere Farms sweet potatoes, peeled and cut into 3cm balls
- 400ml tin Isle Sun Coconut-milk
- 1/2 vegetable stock block, created as much as 300ml
- 200g Grower's Harvest long-grain rice
- 300g frozen green beans
- 150g Red Mere Farms lettuce
- 1 Sun trail Farms lemon, 1/2 juiced, 1/2 cut into wedges to function

DIRECTIONS

1. Set the onion, ginger, garlic, coriander stalks tikka powder along with half of the cashew nuts in a food processor. Insert 2 tablespoons of water and blitz to a chunky paste.
2. In a large skillet, warm the oil over moderate heat. Insert the paste and cook, stirring for 5 minutes. Bring the sweet potatoes, stir, and then pour into the coconut milk and stock. Bring to the simmer and boil for 25-35 minutes before the sweet potatoes are tender.
3. Meanwhile, cook the rice pack directions. Toast the rest of the cashews in a dry skillet.
4. Stir the beans into the curry and then simmer for two minutes. Insert the lettuce in handfuls, allowing each to simmer before adding the following; simmer for 1 minute. Bring the lemon juice, to taste, and the majority of the coriander leaves. Scatter on the remaining coriander and cashews, then use the rice and lemon wedges.

Nutritions: *Power 2290 kj (544 kcal) (27%), Fat 20 g (28%), Saturates 8 g (41%) Sugars 14 g (15%)*

48. CHICKEN LIVER ALONG WITH TOMATO RAGU RECIPE

INGREDIENTS

- 2 tablespoons olive oil
- 1 onion, finely chopped
- 2 carrots scrubbed and simmer
- 4 garlic cloves, finely chopped
- 1/4 x 30g pack fresh ginger, stalks finely chopped, leaves ripped
- 380g package poultry livers, finely chopped, and almost any sinew removed and lost
- 400g tin Grower's Harvest chopped berries
- 1 chicken stock cube, created around 300ml
- 1/2 teaspoon caster sugar
- 300g penne
- 1/4 Sun trail Farms lemon, juiced

DIRECTIONS

1. Heat 1 tablespoon oil in a large skillet, over a low-medium heating system. Fry the onion and carrots for 10 minutes, stirring periodically. Stir in the ginger and garlic pops and cook 2 minutes more. Transfer into a bowl set aside.
2. Twist the pan into high heat and then add the oil. Bring the chicken livers and simmer for 5 minutes until browned. Pour the onion mix to the pan and then stir in the tomatoes, sugar, and stock. Season, bring to the boil, and then simmer for 20 minutes until reduced and thickened and also the liver is cooked through. Meanwhile, cook pasta to package direction.
3. Taste the ragu and put in a second pinch of sugar more seasoning, if needed. Put in a squeeze of lemon juice to taste and stir in two of the ripped basil leaves. Divide the pasta between four bowls, then spoon across the ragu and top with the rest of the basil.

Nutritions: *Power 1980 kj (469 kcal) (23%), Fat 12 g (17%), Saturates 2 g (11%) Sugars 12 g (13%)*

49. MINTED LAMB WITH A COUSCOUS SALAD RECIPE

INGREDIENTS

- 75g couscous
- 1/2 chicken stock block, composed to 125ml
- 30g pack refreshing flat-leaf parsley, sliced
- 3 mint sprigs, leaves picked and sliced
- 1 tablespoon olive oil
- 200g pack suspended BBQ minted lamb leg beans, de-frosted
- 200g lettuce berries, sliced
- 1/4 teaspoon, sliced
- 1 spring onion, sliced
- Pinch of ground cumin
- 1/2 lemon, zested and juiced
- 50g reduced-fat salad cheese

DIRECTIONS

1. Place the couscous into a heatproof bowl and then pour on the inventory. Cover and set aside for 10 minutes, then fluff with a fork and stir in the herbs.
2. Meanwhile, rub a little oil within the lamb steaks and season. Cook to package direction, then slit.
3. Mix the tomatoes, cucumber and spring onion into the couscous with the oil, the cumin, and lemon juice and zest. Crumble on the salad and serve with the bunny.

Nutritions: *Power 1945 kj (463 kcal) (23%), Fat 19 g (27%), Saturates 8 g (38%) Sugars 11 g (12%)*

50. JACKFRUIT TORTILLA BOWLS RECIPE

INGREDIENTS

- 2 sweet corn cobbetts
- 1 red chili, finely chopped
- 2 teaspoons olive oil
- 1 lime, juiced
- 15g fresh coriander, chopped, plus extra to garnish
- 150g package stained jackfruit in tex-mex sauce
- 210g tin kidney beans, drained
- 125g roasted red peppers (in the jar), drained and chopped
- 2 whitened tortilla packs
- 1/2 round lettuce, ripped

DIRECTIONS

1. Heat a griddle pan on a high temperature (or light a barbecue). Griddle the cobettes 10-12 minutes, turning until cooked and charred throughout. Remove from the pan and also stand upright onto a plank.
2. Use a sharp knife to carefully reduce the span of this corn, staying near to the heart, to clear away the kernels. Mix that the kernels with the eucalyptus oil, half of the carrot juice along with half an hour of the coriander.
3. Heat the jackfruit and sauce in a saucepan with the legumes, peppers, staying lime, coriander, and juice on medium-low heating for 3-4 minutes until heated through; now.
4. Griddle the wraps for 10-20 seconds each side to char. Tear into pieces and serve together with all the jackfruit lettuce and sweet corn salsa.

Nutritions: *Power 1485 kj (354 kcal) (18%), Fat 10 g (14%), Saturates 1 g (7%) Sugars 10 g (11%)*

51. CARROT, COURGETTE AND HALLOUMI HAMBURGERS

INGREDIENTS

- 1 big carrot, grated
- 1 large courgette, grated
- 225g halloumi, grated
- 2 spring onions, finely chopped
- 90g bread crumbs
- 1 tablespoon ground cumin
- 1 tablespoon ground coriander
- 1/2 teaspoon salt
- 2 tablespoons
- 2 tablespoons flour
- 4 brioche buns, halved
- 50g baby spinach leaves
- 1 big tomato, sliced
- 1 small red onion, chopped
- 1/2 pineapple, peeled into ribbons
- Tzatziki, to function

DIRECTIONS

1. Place the courgette into a clean tea towel and squeeze to eradicate any liquid. Hint into a big bowl and then add the carrot, halloumi, onion, bread crumbs, cumin, coriander, eggs, salt, and flour. Stir well to mix.
2. Put simply over half the mix in a food processor and pulse until the mixture starts to stay. Reunite back this into the booked mix and mix well.
3. Divide the mix into 4 and then form patties. Heat a grill or griddle pan into a moderate heat. Cook the hamburgers for 45 minutes each side until golden and cooked through.
4. Insert the hamburger buns into the grill till lightly toasted. To assemble the burgers, put lettuce leaves on the base of each bun. Top with the hamburger, a piece of tomato, pineapple ribbon along with a spoonful of tzatziki.

Nutritions: *Calories 523, Power 523 kcal (26%), Fat 24 g (34%), Saturates 12 g (62%), Sugars 12 g (13%)*

52. RITA'S 'ROWDY' ENCHILADAS

INGREDIENTS

- 2 large chicken breasts (about 400g)
- 2 red peppers, thinly chopped
- 1 tablespoon olive oil
- 3/4 teaspoons mild chili powder
- 1 teaspoon 1/2 teaspoons ground cumin
- 3/4 teaspoons smoked paprika
- 80g grated mozzarella
- 8 plain tortilla wraps
- 65g ripe cheddar, grated
- 10g fresh coriander, roughly sliced
- The sauce
- 1 tablespoon olive oil
- 1/2 onion, finely chopped
- 2 teaspoons cloves, crushed
- 500g tomato paste
- 1 tablespoon chipotle chili paste
- 400g tin black beans drained and rinsed
- 1/2 lime, juiced

Nutritions: *Power 3185 kj (757 kcal) (38%), Fat 24 g (35%) Saturates 10 g (51%) Sugars 14 g (15%)*

DIRECTIONS

1. Preheat the oven to gas 5, 190°C, buff 170°C. Set the chicken in a 20 x 30cm skillet with all the pepper, olive oil, chili powder, cumin, and paprika. Mix to coat, then cover with foil. Roast for 25-30 minutes before the chicken is cooked and tender with no pink meat remains. Take out the chicken from the dish and then shred with two forks. Reserve in a bowl.
2. Meanwhile, make the sauce. Heat the oil in a saucepan on a low heat and cook the garlic and onion for 10 minutes. Stir from the paste and chipotle chili glue; increase heat to moderate, bring to a simmer and cook for a further 10 minutes, stirring periodically. Bring the beans and carrot juice season.
3. Mix one-third of this sauce plus half of the mozzarella to the cultured broccoli and chicken.
4. To gather, spoon 4 tablespoons of this sauce in exactly the same baking dish before. Spoon a bit of the chicken mixture down the middle of each tortilla, roll up, and then put it from the dish. Repeat with the tortillas and filling, then place them alongside in order that they do not shatter.
5. Pour the remaining sauce on the top and then scatter within the cheddar and remaining mozzarella. Bake in the oven for 20-25 minutes until the cheese has melted and begun to brownish. Scatter together with all the coriander to function.

Freezing and defrosting recommendations

6. Cook as educated and let it cool completely. Subsequently, move to an airtight, freezer-safe container, seal, and freeze up to 1-3 weeks. Guarantee the meatballs are underwater in the sauce since they are going to freeze far better.
7. To serve, defrost thoroughly in the refrigerator overnight before reheating. Put in a bowl over moderate heat, stirring occasionally until the dish is heated throughout.

53. FULL-OF-VEG HASH RECIPE

INGREDIENTS

- 750g potatoes, pared and grated
- 2 tablespoons olive oil
- 100g streaky bacon, roughly sliced
- 2 red onions, finely chopped
- 300g carrots, peeled and diced
- 2 courgettes, diced
- 2 garlic cloves, crushed
- 4 eggs
- 5g refreshing flat-leaf parsley, sliced
- 1 red chili, chopped (optional)
- 1/2 x 340g jar pickled red cabbage

DIRECTIONS

1. Preheat the oven to 220°C, buff 200°C. Bring a bowl of soapy water to the boil and then simmer the potatoes for 5 minutes, then drain and put aside.
2. Heat 1 tablespoon oil in a large, ovenproof skillet on a high heat and fry the bacon for 5 minutes until crispy. Add the carrots, onions, courgettes, onions, and garlic; season and then cook for 5 minutes. Transfer the pan into the oven and bake for 25-30 minutes before the vegetables are tender and gold.
3. Meanwhile, heat the remaining oil in a skillet on medium-high heating and fry the eggs 2-3 minutes or until cooked to your liking.
4. Split the hash between two plates and top each with lettuce. Scatter with parsley and simmer, then function with the pickled red cabbage onto both.

Nutritions: *Calories 387, Power 1620 kj (387 kcal) (19%), Fat 17 g (25%) Saturates 4 g (22%), Sugars 11 g (13%)*

54. BACON AND EGG FRIED RICE RECIPE

INGREDIENTS

- 350g long-grain rice, well rinsed
- 1 1/2 tablespoon olive oil
- 100g streaky bacon, diced
- 2 peppers, finely chopped
- 2 red onions, finely chopped
- 200g carrots, peeled and coarsely grated
- 2 garlic cloves, crushed
- 5cm slice ginger, peeled and grated
- 1 red chili, finely chopped (optional)
- 2 eggs
- 2 teaspoons soy sauce

DIRECTIONS

1. Cook the rice in a big bowl of warm water for 10 minutes until not quite tender. Drain, rinse with warm water and drain. Set aside.
2. Meanwhile, warm 1/2 tablespoon oil in a skillet on a high heat and fry the bacon for 5-7 minutes until golden and crispy. Remove from the pan using a slotted spoon and place aside. Add 1 tablespoon oil and fry the peppers for 10 minutes until lightly bubbling. Add the carrots, onions, ginger, garlic, and chili and fry over a moderate-high temperature for 5 minutes more.
3. Insert the rice and bacon and simmer for 5 minutes, stirring often. Push the rice mix to a single side of this pan and then crack the eggs to the gap. Beat the eggs with a wooden spoon, and then stir throughout the rice. Cook for 2 minutes, then add the soy sauce and then remove from heat. Split between 4 shallow bowls to function.

Nutritions: *Calories 506, Fat 13 g (19%), Saturates 4 g (19%), Sugars 12 g (13%)*

55. SUPER-SPEEDY PRAWN RISOTTO

INGREDIENTS

- 100g diced onion
- 2 x 250g packs whole-grain rice & quinoa
- 200g frozen garden peas
- 2 x 150g packs cooked and peeled king prawns
- 1/285g tote water-cress

DIRECTIONS

1. Heat 1 tablespoon coconut oil in a skillet on medium-high heat and then put in 100g diced onion; cook for 5 minutes. Insert 2 x 250g packs whole-grain rice & quinoa along with 175ml hot vegetable stock (or plain water); together side 200g suspended Garden Peas.
2. Gently split using rice using a wooden spoon. Cover and cook 3 minutes, stirring occasionally, you can add two x 150g packs Cooked and Peeled King Prawns. Cook for 12 minutes before prawns, peas, and rice have been piping hot, and the majority of the liquid was consumed. Remove from heat. Chop 1/2 x 85g tote water-cress and stir throughout; up to taste. Top with watercress leaves and pepper to function.

Nutritions: *Calories 456, Protein 5 g, Carbohydrate 23 g, Fat 6 g)*

56. MISO MARINATED COD WITH STIR-FRIED GREENS AND SESAME

INGREDIENTS

- 1 x 7 ounce skinless cod fillet
- 1 tablespoon mirin
- 3 ½ teaspoon miso
- ¾ cup kale, roughly chopped
- 1 tablespoon extra-virgin olive oil
- 1/8 cup red onion, sliced
- 3/8 cup celery, sliced
- ¼ cup, buckwheat
- 1 bird's eye chili, finely chopped
- 1 garlic clove, finely chopped
- 1 teaspoon finely chopped fresh ginger
- 1 teaspoon sesame seeds
- 3/8 cup green beans
- 2 tablespoon parsley, roughly chopped
- 1 tablespoon tamari
- 1 teaspoon ground turmeric

DIRECTIONS

1. Add one teaspoon of oil, the mirin and miso into a bowl and mix together. Rub the mixture all over the cod and leave it for 30 minutes to marinate. Heat your oven to 220°C or 425°F. Bake the cod for approximately ten minutes.
2. Add the remaining oil into a large fry pan or wok over medium heat. Once hot, add the onions and stir-fry for 3 minutes, then add the garlic, celery, green beans, ginger, chili, and kale. Stir and fry until the kale is well cooked and tender. Add a little water to the pan if needed to aid the cooking process.
3. Cook the buckwheat following the instruction on the packet, add the turmeric three minutes before the end.
4. Add the sesame seeds, tamari, and parsley to the stir fry. Serve with the fish and the greens.

Nutritions: *Calories 213, Fat 4 g, Protein 9 g*

57. BULGUR APPETIZER SALAD

INGREDIENTS

- 1 cup Bulgur
- 2 cups hot water
- Black pepper to the taste
- 2 cups corn
- 1 cucumber, chopped
- 2 tablespoons lemon juice
- 2 tablespoons balsamic vinegar
- ¼ cup olive oil

DIRECTIONS

1. In a bowl, mix Bulgur with the water, cover, leave aside for 30 minutes, fluff with a fork, and transfer to a salad bowl.
2. Add corn, cucumber, oil with lemon juice, vinegar and pepper, toss, divide into small cups and serve.

Nutritions: *Calories 57, Fat 1.3 g, Carbohydrates 10 g, Protein 5 g*

58. COCOA BARS

INGREDIENTS

- 1 cup unsweetened cocoa chips
- 2 cups rolled oats
- 1 cup low-fat peanut butter
- ½ cup chia seeds
- ½ cup raisins
- ¼ cup coconut sugar
- ½ cup coconut milk

DIRECTIONS

1. Put 1 and ½ cups oats in your blender, pulse well, transfer this to a bowl, add the rest of the oats, cocoa chips, chia seeds, raisins, sugar and milk.
2. Stir really well; spread this into a square pan, press well, keep in the fridge for 2 hours, slice into 12 bars and serve.

Nutritions: *Calories 198, Fat 5 g, Fiber 4 g, Carbs 10 g, Protein 89 g*

59. CINNAMON APPLE CHIPS

INGREDIENTS

- Cooking spray
- 2 teaspoons cinnamon powder
- 2 apples, cored and thinly sliced

DIRECTIONS

1. Arrange apple slices on a lined baking sheet, spray them with cooking oil, sprinkle cinnamon, introduce in the oven and bake at 300°F for 2 hours.
2. Divide into bowls and serve as a snack.

Nutritions: *Calories 57, Fat 1.3 g, Carbohydrates 10 g, Protein 5 g*

PREPARATION: 10 MIN   **COOKING: 0 MIN**   **SERVES: 4**

60. GREEK PARTY DIP

INGREDIENTS

- ½ cup coconut cream
- 1 cup fat-free Greek yogurt
- 2 teaspoons dill, dried
- 2 teaspoons thyme, dried
- 1 teaspoon sweet paprika
- 2 teaspoons no-salt-added sun-dried tomatoes, chopped
- 2 teaspoons parsley, chopped
- 2 teaspoons chives, chopped
- Black pepper to the taste

DIRECTIONS

1. In a bowl, mix cream with yogurt, dill with thyme, paprika, tomatoes, parsley, chives and pepper.
2. Stir well, divide into smaller bowls and serve as a dip.

Nutritions: *Calories 100, Fat 1 g, Fiber 4 g, Carbs 8 g, Protein 3 g*

61. SPICY PUMPKIN SEEDS BOWLS

INGREDIENTS

- ½ tablespoon chili powder
- ½ teaspoon cayenne pepper
- 2 cups pumpkin seeds
- 2 teaspoons lime juice

DIRECTIONS

1. Spread pumpkin seeds on a lined baking sheet; add lime juice, cayenne and chili powder.
2. Toss well, introduce in the oven, roast at 275°F for 20 minutes, divide into small bowls and serve as a snack.

Nutritions: *Calories 170, Fat 2 g, Fiber 7 g, Carbs 12 g, Protein 6 g*

PREPARATION: 10 MIN   **COOKING: 0 MIN**   **SERVES: 4**

62. APPLE AND PECANS BOWLS

INGREDIENTS

- 4 big apples, cored, peeled and cubed
- 2 teaspoons lemon juice
- ¼ cup pecans, chopped

DIRECTIONS

1. In a bowl, mix apples with lemon juice and pecans.
2. Toss, divide into small bowls and serve as a snack.

Nutritions: *Calories 120, Fat 4 g, Fiber 3 g, Carbs 12 g, Protein 3 g*

63. SHRIMP MUFFINS

INGREDIENTS

- 1 spaghetti squash, peeled and halved
- 2 tablespoons avocado mayonnaise
- 1 cup low-fat mozzarella cheese, shredded
- 8 ounces shrimp, peeled, cooked and chopped
- 1 and ½ cups almond flour
- 1 teaspoon parsley, dried
- 1 garlic clove, minced
- Black pepper to the taste
- Cooking spray

DIRECTIONS

1. Arrange the squash on a lined baking sheet, introduce in the oven at 375°F, bake for 30 minutes.
2. Scrape flesh into a bowl, add pepper, parsley flakes, flour, shrimp, mayo and mozzarella and stir well.
3. Divide this mix into a muffin tray greased with cooking spray, bake in the oven at 375° F for 15 minutes and serve them cold as a snack.

Nutritions: *Calories 140, Fat 2 g, Fiber 4 g, Carbs 14 g, Protein 12 g*

64. CHEESY MUSHROOMS CAPS

INGREDIENTS

- 20 white mushroom caps
- 1 garlic clove, minced
- 3 tablespoons parsley, chopped
- 2 yellow onions, chopped
- Black pepper to the taste
- ½ cup low-fat parmesan, grated
- ¼ cup low-fat mozzarella, grated
- A drizzle of olive oil
- 2 tablespoons non-fat yogurt

DIRECTIONS

1. Heat up a pan with some oil over medium heat, add garlic and onion, stir, cook for 10 minutes and transfer to a bowl.
2. Add black pepper, garlic, parsley, mozzarella, parmesan and yogurt, stir well.
3. Stuff the mushroom caps with this mix, arrange them on a lined baking sheet, bake in the oven at 400 degrees F for 20 minutes and serve them as an appetizer.

Nutritions: *Calories 120, Fat 1 g, Fiber 3 g, Carbs 11 g, Protein 7 g*

65. MOZZARELLA CAULIFLOWER BARS

INGREDIENTS

- 1 big cauliflower head, riced
- ½ cup low-fat mozzarella cheese, shredded
- ¼ cup egg whites
- 1 teaspoon Italian seasoning
- Black pepper to the taste

DIRECTIONS

1. Spread the cauliflower rice on a lined baking sheet, cook in the oven at 375 degrees F for 20 minutes, transfer to a bowl, add black pepper, cheese, seasoning and egg whites, stir well, spread into a rectangle pan and press well on the bottom.
2. Introduce in the oven at 375°F, bake for 20 minutes, cut into 12 bars and serve as a snack.

Nutritions: *Calories 140, Fat 1 g, Fiber 3 g, Carbs 6 g, Protein 6 g*

66. SHRIMP AND PINEAPPLE SALSA

INGREDIENTS

- 1-pound large shrimp, peeled and deveined
- 20 ounces canned pineapple chunks
- 1 tablespoon garlic powder
- 1 cup red bell peppers, chopped
- Black pepper to the taste

DIRECTIONS

1. Place shrimp in a baking dish, add pineapple, garlic, bell peppers and black pepper.
2. Toss a bit, introduce in the oven, bake at 375°F for 40 minutes, divide into small bowls and serve cold.

Nutritions: *Calories 170, Fat 5 g, Fiber 4 g, Carbs 15 g, Protein 11 g*

67. STRAWBERRY BUCKWHEAT PANCAKES

INGREDIENTS

- 100g (3½ ounces) strawberries, chopped
- 100g (3½ ounces) buckwheat flour
- 1 egg
- 250mls (8 fluid ounces) milk
- 1 teaspoon olive oil
- 1 teaspoon olive oil for frying
- Freshly squeezed juice of 1 orange
- 175 calories per serving

DIRECTIONS

1. Pour the milk into a bowl and mix in the egg and a teaspoon of olive oil. Sift in the flour to the liquid mixture until smooth and creamy. Allow it to rest for 15 minutes.
2. Heat a little oil in a pan and pour in a quarter of the mixture (or to the size you prefer).
3. Sprinkle in a quarter of the strawberries into the batter—cook for around 2 minutes on each side. Serve hot with a drizzle of orange juice. You could try experimenting with other berries such as blueberries and blackberries.

Nutritions: *Calories 254, Fat 21 g, Carbs 25 g, Protein 8 g*

68. STRAWBERRY & NUT GRANOLA

INGREDIENTS

- 200g (7 ounces) oats
- 250g (9 ounces) buckwheat flakes
- 100g (3½ ounces) walnuts, chopped
- 100g (3½ ounces) almonds, chopped
- 100g (3½ ounces) dried strawberries
- 1½ teaspoons ground ginger
- 1½ teaspoons ground cinnamon
- 120mls (4 fluid ounces) olive oil
- 2 tablespoons honey

DIRECTIONS

1. Combine the oats, buckwheat flakes, nuts, ginger and cinnamon. In a saucepan, warm the oil and honey. Stir until the honey has melted.
2. Pour the warm oil into the dry ingredients and mix well. Spread the mixture out on a large baking tray (or two) and bake in the oven at 150°C (300°F) for around 50 minutes until the granola is golden. Allow it to cool.
3. Add in the dried berries. Store in an airtight container until ready to use. Can be served with yogurt, milk or even dry as a handy snack.

Nutritions: *Calories 391, Fat 0 g, Fiber 6 g, Carbs 3 g, Protein 8 g*

69. FRUIT & NUT YOGURT CRUNCH

INGREDIENTS

- 100g (3½ ounces) plain Greek yogurt
- 50g (2 ounces) strawberries, chopped
- 6 walnut halves, chopped
- Sprinkling of cocoa powder

DIRECTIONS

1. Stir half of the chopped strawberries into the yogurt.
2. Using a glass, place a layer of yogurt with a sprinkling of strawberries and walnuts, followed by another layer of the same until you reach the top of the glass.
3. Garnish with walnuts pieces and a dusting of cocoa powder.

Nutritions: *Calories 296, Fat 4 g, Fiber 2 g, Carbs 5 g, Protein 9 g*

PREPARATION: 5 MIN   COOKING: 15 MIN   SERVES: 4

70. CHEESY BAKED EGGS

INGREDIENTS

- 4 large eggs
- 75g (3 ounces) cheese, grated
- 25g (1 ounce) fresh rocket (arugula) leaves, finely chopped
- 1 tablespoon parsley
- ½ teaspoon ground turmeric
- 1 tablespoon olive oil

DIRECTIONS

1. Grease each ramekin dish with a little olive oil. Divide the rocket (arugula) between the ramekin dishes, then break an egg into each one.
2. Sprinkle a little parsley and turmeric on top, then sprinkle on the cheese. Place the ramekins in a preheated oven at 220°C/425°F for 15 minutes, until the eggs are set and the cheese is bubbling.

Nutritions: *Calories 198, Fat 9 g, Fiber 3 g, Carbs 2 g, Protein 13 g*

71. GREEN EGG SCRAMBLE

INGREDIENTS

- 2 eggs, whisked
- 25g (1 ounce) rocket (arugula) leaves
- 1 teaspoon chives, chopped
- 1 teaspoon fresh basil, chopped
- 1 teaspoon fresh parsley, chopped
- 1 tablespoon olive oil

DIRECTIONS

1. Mix the eggs together with the rocket (arugula) and herbs.
2. Heat the oil in a frying pan and pour in the egg mixture.
3. Gently stir until it's lightly scrambled. Season and serve.

Nutritions: *Calories 250, Fat 5 g, Fiber 7 g, Carbs 8 g, Protein 11 g*

PREPARATION: 10 MIN   COOKING: 5 MIN   SERVES: 8

72. COURGETTE RISOTTO

INGREDIENTS

- 2 tablespoons olive oil
- 4 cloves garlic, finely chopped
- 1.5 pounds Arborio rice
- 6 tomatoes, chopped
- 2 teaspoons chopped rosemary
- 6 courgettes, finely diced
- 1 ¼ cups peas, fresh or frozen
- 12 cups hot vegetable stock
- 1 cup chopped
- Salt to taste
- Freshly ground pepper

DIRECTIONS

1. Place a large, heavy-bottomed pan over medium heat. Add oil. When the oil is heated, add onion and sauté until translucent.
2. Stir in the tomatoes and cook until soft.
3. Next, stir in the rice and rosemary. Mix well.
4. Add half the stock and cook until dry. Stir frequently.
5. Add remaining stock and cook for 3-4 minutes.
6. Add courgette and peas and cook until rice is tender. Add salt and pepper to taste.
7. Stir in the basil. Let it sit for 5 minutes.

Nutritions: *Calories 406, Fats 5 g, Carbohydrates 82 g, Proteins 14 g*

73. BROWN BASMATI RICE PILAF

INGREDIENTS

- ½ tablespoon vegan butter
- ½ cup mushrooms, chopped
- ½ cup brown basmati rice
- 2-3 tablespoons water
- 1/8 teaspoon dried thyme
- Ground pepper to taste
- ½ tablespoon olive oil
- ¼ cup green onion, chopped
- 1 cup vegetable broth
- ¼ teaspoon salt
- ¼ cup chopped, toasted pecans

DIRECTIONS

1. Place a saucepan over medium-low heat. Add butter and oil.
2. When it melts, add mushrooms and cook until slightly tender.
3. Stir in the green onion and brown rice—cook for 3 minutes. Stir constantly.
4. Stir in the broth, water, salt and thyme.
5. When it begins to boil, lower heat and cover with a lid. Simmer until rice is cooked. Add more water or broth if required.
6. Stir in the pecans and pepper.
7. Serve.

Nutritions: *Calories 189, Fats 11 g, Carbohydrates 19 g, Proteins 4 g*

74. SIRTFOOD DIET'S SHAKSHUKA

INGREDIENTS

- 1 tablespoon chopped parsley
- 1 teaspoon extra virgin olive oil
- 1 teaspoon paprika
- ½ cup red onion, finely chopped
- 30g kale, stems removed and roughly chopped
- 1 garlic clove, finely chopped
- 30g celery, finely chopped
- 1 bird's eye chili, finely chopped
- 1 teaspoon ground turmeric
- 1 teaspoon ground cumin
- 2 cups tinned chopped tomatoes
- 2 medium eggs

DIRECTIONS

1. Place a small, deep-sided fry pan over medium-low heat. Add the oil once hot, and then add the chili, spices, celery, garlic, and onions. Fry for about 2 minutes.
2. Add the tomatoes, and then allow the sauce to simmer gently for approximately 20 minutes while stirring frequently.
3. Add the kale to the pot and cook for another five minutes. Add a little water if the sauce gets too thick. Stir in the parsley once the sauce becomes nicely creamy.
4. Create two little wells in the sauce, and then break each egg into the wells. Reduce your heat to the lowest and cover the pan with a foil or with its lid. Allow the eggs to cook for about 10 minutes or until the whites are firm and the yolks remain runny. Cook for another four minutes if you want the yolks to be firm.
5. Serve immediately.

Nutritions: *Calories 657, Protein 87 g, Fat 4 g, Sugar 6 g*

75. THE SIRTFOOD'S WALNUT AND DATE PORRIDGE

INGREDIENTS

- ½ cup strawberries, hulled
- 200ml milk or dairy-free alternative
- ½ cup buckwheat flakes
- 1 medjool date, chopped
- Walnut butter - 1 teaspoon, or chopped walnut halves

DIRECTIONS

1. Place the date and the milk in a pan, heat gently before adding the buckwheat flakes. Then cook until the porridge gets to your desired consistency.
2. Add the walnuts, stir, then top with the strawberries.
3. Serve.

Nutritions: *Calories 254, Protein 65 g, Fat 4 g, Vitamin B*

76. VIETNAMESE TURMERIC FISH WITH MANGO AND HERBS SAUCE

INGREDIENTS

For the fish:

- 2 tablespoons coconut oil to fry the fish
- 1 ¼ pounds fresh codfish, skinless and boneless—(cut into 2-inch piece wide)
- Pinch of sea salt, to taste

Fish marinade:

Marinate the fish for a minimum of one hour or overnight.
- 1 tablespoon Chinese cooking wine
- 1 tablespoon turmeric powder
- 1 teaspoon sea salt
- 2 tablespoons olive oil
- 2 teaspoons minced ginger

Mango Dipping Sauce:

- Juice of ½ lime
- 1 medium-sized ripe mango
- 2 tablespoons rice vinegar
- 1 teaspoon dry red chili pepper (stir in before serving)
- 1 garlic clove

Infused scallion and dill oil

- 2 cups fresh dill
- 2 cups scallions (slice into long thin shape)
- A pinch of sea salt, to taste

Toppings:

- Nuts (pine or cashew nuts)
- Lime juice (as much as you like)
- Fresh cilantro (as much as you like)
  A pinch of sea salt, to taste

DIRECTIONS

1. Add all the ingredients under "Mango Dipping Sauce" into your food processor. Blend until you get your preferred consistency.

Pan-fry the fish:

2. Add two tablespoons of coconut oil in a large non-stick fry pan and heat over high heat. Once hot, add the pre-marinated fish. Add the slices of the fish into the pan individually—divide into batches for easy frying, if necessary.
3. Once you hear a loud sizzle, reduce the heat to medium-high.
4. Do not move or turn the fish until it turns golden brown on one side; then turn it to the other side to fry, about 5 minutes on each side. Add more coconut oil to the pan if needed—season with the sea salt.

Make the scallion and dill infused oil:

5. Using the remaining oil in the fry pan, set to medium-high heat, add 2 cups of dill, and 2 cups of scallions. Put off the heat after you have added the dill and scallions. Toss them gently for about 15 seconds, until the dill and scallions have wilted. Add a dash of sea salt to season.
6. Pour the dill, scallion, and infused oil over the fish. Serve with mango dipping sauce, nuts, lime, and fresh cilantro.

Nutritions: *Calories 234, Fat 23 g, Protein 76 g, Sugar 5 g*

77. SIRTFOOD CHICKEN AND KALE CURRY

INGREDIENTS

- 250ml boiling water
- 7 ounces skinless and boneless chicken thighs
- 2 tablespoons ground turmeric
- 1 tablespoon olive oil
- 1 red onions, diced
- 1 bird's eye chili, finely chopped
- ½ tablespoon freshly chopped ginger
- ½ tablespoon curry powder
- 1 ½ cloves garlic, crushed
- 1 cardamom pods
- ½ tin chopped tomatoes
- 100ml tinned coconut milk, light
- 2 cups chicken stock
- 1 cup tinned chopped tomatoes

DIRECTIONS

1. Place the chicken thighs in a non-metallic bowl; add one tablespoon of turmeric and one teaspoon of olive oil. Mix together and keep aside to marinate for approximately 30 minutes.
2. Fry the chicken thighs over medium heat for about 5 minutes until well cooked and brown on all sides. Remove from the pan and set aside.
3. Add the remaining oil into a fry pan on medium heat. Then add the onion, ginger, garlic, and chili. Fry for about 10 minutes until soft.
4. Add one tablespoon of the turmeric and half tablespoon of curry powder to the pan and cook for another 2 minutes.
5. Then add the cardamom pods, coconut milk, tomatoes, and chicken stock. Allow simmering for thirty minutes.
6. Add the chicken once the sauce has reduced a little in the pan, followed by the kale. Cook until the kale is tender and the chicken is warm enough.
7. Serve with buckwheat.
8. Garnish with the chopped coriander.

Nutritions: *Calories 313, Protein 13 g, Fat 6 g, Carbohydrate 23 g*

78. MEDITERRANEAN BAKED PENNE

INGREDIENTS

- 1 tablespoon extra-virgin olive oil
- ½ cup fine dry bread crumbs
- 2 small zucchini, chopped
- 1 medium eggplant, chopped
- 1 medium onion, chopped
- 1 red bell pepper, seeded and chopped
- 1 celery stalk, sliced
- 1 garlic clove, minced
- Salt and freshly ground pepper to taste
- ¼ cup dry white wine
- 1 x 28-ounce plum tomatoes, drained and coarsely chopped, juice reserved
- 2 tablespoons freshly grated Parmesan cheese
- 2 large eggs, lightly beaten
- 1 ½ cups coarsely grated part-skim mozzarella cheese
- 1 pound dried penne rig ate or rigatoni

DIRECTIONS

1. Preheat your oven to 375°F. Apply nonstick spray on a 3-quart baking dish. Then coat the dish with ¼ cup of bread crumbs, tapping out the excess.
2. Heat the oil in a large non-stick skillet over medium-high heat. Then add the onion, celery, bell pepper, eggplant, and zucchini. Cook for about 10 minutes, stirring occasionally, until smooth. Then add the garlic and cook for another minute. Add the wine, stir and cook for about 2 minutes, long enough for the wine to almost evaporate, then add the juice and tomatoes. Bring to a simmer and cook for about 10 to 15 minutes, until thickened, season with pepper and salt. Transfer to a large bowl and allow cooling.
3. Pour water into a pot, add some salt, and then allow boiling. Add the penne into the boiling salted water to cook for about 10 minutes, until al dente. Drain and rinse the pasta under running water. Toss the pasta with the vegetable mixture, and then stir in the mozzarella.
4. Scoop the pasta mixture and place into the prepared baking dish. Drizzle the broken eggs evenly over the top. Mix the Parmesan and ¼ cups of breadcrumbs in a small bowl and then sprinkle evenly over the top of the dish.
5. Place the dish into the oven to bake for about 40 to 50 minutes, until bubbly and golden.
6. Allow to stand for 10 min before you serve.

Nutritions: *Calories 372, Protein 45 g, Fat 8 g, Sugar 2 g*

79. PRAWN ARRABBIATA

INGREDIENTS

- 1 cup raw or cooked prawns
- 1 tablespoon extra-virgin olive oil
- ½ cup buckwheat pasta

For Arrabbiata Sauce

- 1 tablespoon chopped parsley
- ¼ cup celery, finely chopped
- 2 cups tinned chopped tomatoes
- 1/3 cup red onion, finely chopped
- 1 garlic clove, finely chopped
- 1 teaspoon extra virgin olive oil
- 1 teaspoon dried mixed herbs
- 1 bird's eye chili, finely chopped
- 2 tablespoons white wine (optional)

DIRECTIONS

1. Add the olive oil into your fry-pan and fry the dried herbs, celery, and onions over medium-low heat for about two minutes. Increase heat to medium, add the wine, and cook for another one min. Add the tomatoes to the pan and allow simmering for about 30 minutes, over medium-low heat, until you get a nice creamy consistency. Add a little water if the sauce gets too thick.
2. While the sauce is cooking, cook the pasta following the instruction on the packet. Drain the water once the pasta is done cooking, toss with the olive oil and set aside until needed.
3. If using raw prawns, add them to your sauce and cook for another four minutes, until the prawns turn opaque and pink, then add the parsley. If using cooked prawns, add them at the same time with the parsley and allow the sauce to boil.
4. Add the already cooked pasta to the sauce, mix them, and serve.

Nutritions: *Calories 321, Protein 19 g, Fat 2 g*

SALAD RECIPES

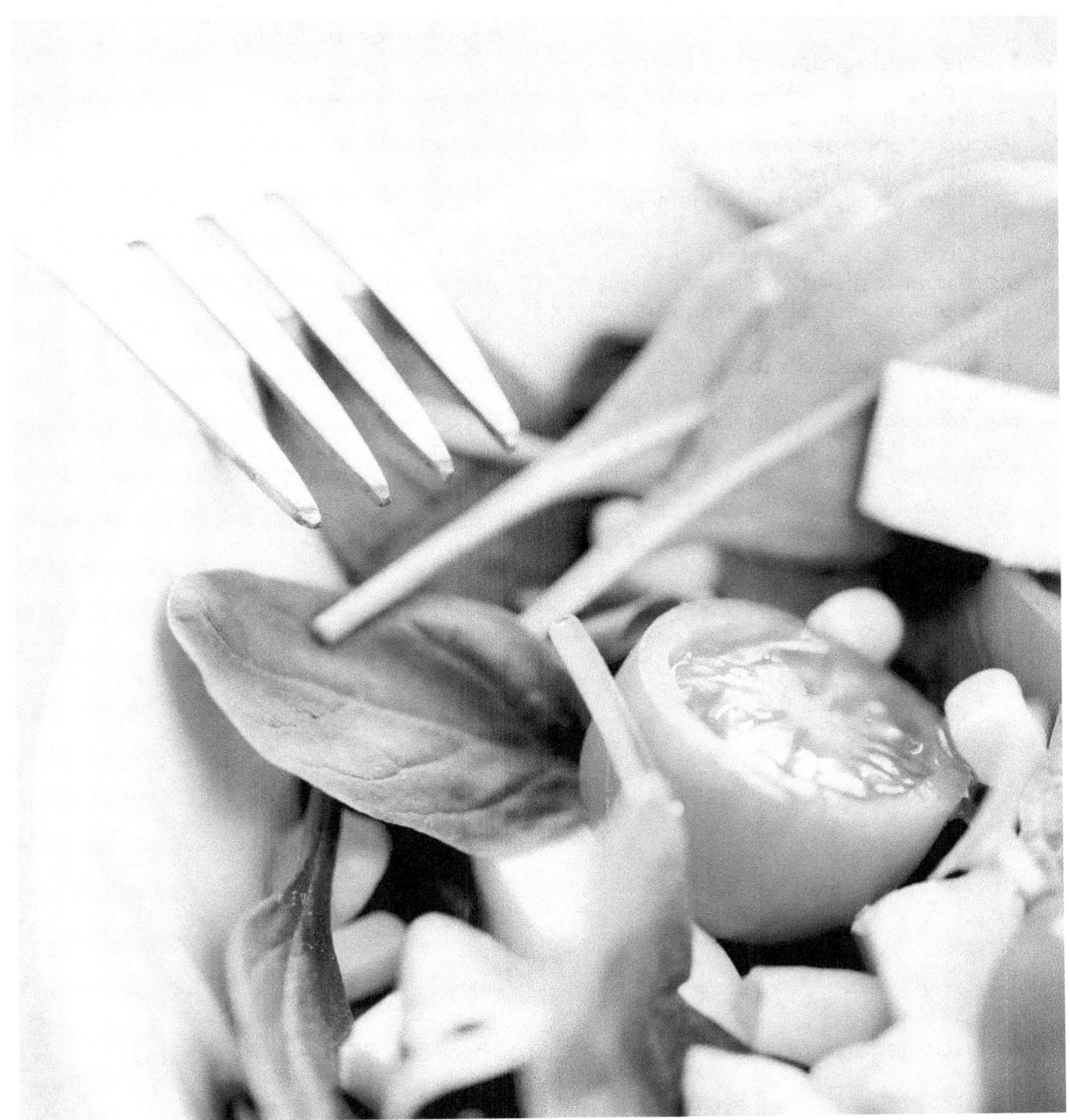

80. WALNUTS AVOCADO SALAD

INGREDIENTS

- ¼ cup of chopped parsley
- ¼ lemon juice
- 1 tablespoon of extra virgin olive oil
- 1 large medjool date, pitted and chopped
- 1 tablespoon of capers
- ⅛ cup of chopped walnuts
- ⅛ cup of sliced red onion
- ½ cup of celery, including leaves, sliced
- ½ cup of avocado, peeled, stoned, and sliced
- 100g of smoked salmon slices (3 ½ ounces)
- 50g of endive leaves (1 ¾ ounces)
- 50g of arugula (1 ¾ ounces)

DIRECTIONS

1. Place the endive leaves, parsley, celery leaves and arugula in a large bowl or plate.
2. Mix together the remaining ingredients and serve over the leaves.

Nutritions: *Calories 89, Sugar 2 g, Carbohydrate 33 gVitamin K and C*

81. POACHED PEAR SALAD WITH DIJON VINEGAR DRESSING

INGREDIENTS

For the dressing:

- 75ml olive oil
- 75ml walnut oil
- 1 tablespoon of red wine vinegar
- 1 tablespoon of Dijon mustard
- Freshly ground Pepper to taste
- Salt to taste
- 1 teaspoon dried mixed herbs
- 1 bird's eye chili, finely chopped
- 2 tablespoons white wine (optional)

For the salad:

- 200g of Gorgonzola cheese, slice finely
- Few rocket leaves
- 100g of Walnuts
- 2 ripe pears (peeled and core) cut into quarters
- 2 bay leaves
- Small bunch of thyme
- 40g of caster sugar
- 180ml of red wine

DIRECTIONS

1. Boil the wine in a saucepan. Along with the bay leaves, sugar and thyme. Simmer over medium-low heat.
2. Add the pear into the simmering liquid and poach for 10 minutes. Remove pan from heat and set aside to cool pears in poaching liquid.
3. In a bowl, whisk together the mustard, salt, vinegar, and pepper until well whisk; slowly stream in the oil and whisking as you add.
4. Arrange salad ingredients on a serving plate and drizzle with the dressing.

Nutritions: *Calories 88, Sugar 4 g, Carbohydrate 24 g*

82. STEAK ARUGULA STRAWBERRY SALAD

INGREDIENTS

Steak:

- 1/2 tablespoon extra-virgin olive oil
- Montreal steak seasoning
- 2 beef tenderloin steaks

Salad:

- 1/8 cup of slivered walnuts
- 1/4 cup of crumbled feta cheese
- 1/2 cup of sliced strawberries
- 1/2 cup blueberries
- 1/2 cup of raspberries
- 3 cups of arugula
- Balsamic Vinaigrette
- Salt and pepper
- 1/4 teaspoon of Dijon mustard
- 1 1/2 teaspoon of sugar
- 1/8 cup of olive oil
- 1/8 cup of balsamic vinegar

DIRECTIONS

Steak:

1. Run the Montreal steak seasoning all over the steak and let sit for 5-10 minutes.
2. Heat oil over medium-high heat in a cast-iron skillet. Once it's simmering, add in the steak and cook about 5-7 minutes; flip and cook the other side for 3-4 minutes or until it's cooked the way you like your meat.
3. Set steak aside in a plate and let cool for 5 minutes before slicing into strips.

Salad:

4. Combine together the salad ingredients in a large bowl.
5. In a small shaker, add together all vinaigrette ingredients and shake until well mixed. Pour dressing over salad and toss to evenly coat.

To serve:

6. Divide the salad in 2 bowls and top with steak.
7. Notes:
8. You can keep the dressing for up to one week in the fridge.

Nutritions: *Kcal 506, Net carbs 17 g, Fat 37 g, Fiber 5 g, Protein 23 g*

83. SUPER FRUIT SALAD

INGREDIENTS

- 10 blueberries
- 10 red seedless grapes
- 1 apple, cored and chopped roughly
- 1 orange, halved
- 1 teaspoon of honey
- ½ cup of freshly made matcha green tea

DIRECTIONS

1. Combine 1/2 cup green tea with the honey and stir until dissolved, Squeeze in half of the orange into the green tea mix. Leave to cool.
2. Chop the second orange half into pieces and transfer into a bowl. Add in the blueberries, chopped apple and grapes. Pour the cooled tea on top of the salad mix and allow soaking a little before serving.

Nutritions: *Kcal 200, Net carbs 40 g, Fat 1 g, Fiber 5 g, Protein 2 g*

84. SIRTFOOD SALMON LENTILS SALAD

INGREDIENTS

- 20g of sliced red onion
- 40g of sliced celery
- 10g of chopped lovage
- 10g of chopped parsley
- Juice of 1/4 of a lemon
- 1 tablespoon of extra virgin olive oil
- 1 large medjool date, remove pit and chopped
- 1 tablespoon of capers
- 15g of chopped walnuts
- 80g of avocado, peeled, pitted and sliced
- 100g tinned green lentils or cooked Puy lentils
- 50g of chicory leaves
- 50g of rocket

DIRECTIONS

1. On a large plate, add the salad leaves.
2. Mix together the remaining ingredients and spread mixture over leaves to serve.

Nutritions: *Kcal 400, Net carbs 20 g, Fat 25 g, Fiber 14 g, Protein 10 g*

85. BLUEBERRY KALE SALAD WITH GINGER LIME DRESSING

INGREDIENTS

- 3 tablespoons of white wine vinegar
- 1 tablespoon of honey
- 2 tablespoons of finely chopped ginger, crystallized
- 3 tablespoons of lime juice
- Salt and pepper to taste

Salad:

- 1/4 cup of slivered walnuts toasted
- 1/2-3/4 cup of fresh blueberries
- 1/3 thinly sliced red onion
- 8 cups of kale, de-stemmed and chopped into pieces

DIRECTIONS

1. Combine together the entire dressing ingredients in a medium bowl until well mixed.
2. Add sliced onion, chopped kale, toss to coat. Leave to marinate for about 1-4 hours, depending on how much time you have, tossing periodically. This is an important step to remove the bitterness from the kale.
3. Add toasted walnuts and blueberries. Toss to coat.

Nutritions: *Kcal 91, Net carbs 10 g, Fat 3.69 g, Fiber 3 g, Protein 3 g*

86. FANCY CHICKEN SALAD

INGREDIENTS

- 1 bird's eye chili
- 20g of diced red onion
- 1 finely chopped medjool date
- 6 finely chopped Walnut halves
- 100g of cooked chicken breast, chopped into bite-sized chunks
- 1/2 teaspoon of mild curry powder
- 1 teaspoon of ground turmeric
- 1 teaspoon of chopped Coriander
- Juice of 1/4 of a lemon
- 75g of natural yogurt
- 40g of rocket

DIRECTIONS

1. In a bowl, mix together the lemon juice, yogurt, spices and coriander. Mix in the other ingredients until well blended.
2. Serve over a bed of the rocket.

Nutritions: *(Natural yogurt not included), Kcal 340, Net carbs 22 g, Fat 13 g Fiber 5 g, Protein 36 g*

87. OLIVE, TOMATO, YELLOW PEPPER, RED ONION, CUCUMBER SLICES AND FETA SKEWERS

INGREDIENTS

- 100g of feta, cut into 8 cubes
- 100 g of cucumber, cut in quarters and halved
- Half red onion, cut in half and sliced into 8 pieces
- 1 yellow pepper (or any color you like) cut into 8 squares
- 8 cherry tomatoes
- 8 large black olives
- 2 wooden skewers, soaked for 30 minutes in water before use

For dressing:

- ½ crushed clove garlic
- 1 teaspoon of balsamic vinegar
- ½ lemon Juice
- A few finely chopped basil leaves (or ½ teaspoon of dried mixed herbs)
- 1 tablespoon of extra virgin olive oil
- A few leaves, finely chopped oregano (skip this if using dried mixed herbs)
- Freshly ground black pepper
- Salt to taste

DIRECTIONS

1. Pierce each skewer through the olive, tomato, yellow pepper, red onion, cucumber slices and feta. Repeat a second time.
2. Combine the dressing ingredients in a sealable container and mix thoroughly. Pour dressing over the skewers.

Nutritions: *Kcal 228, Net carbs 13 g, Fat 15 g, Fiber 3 g, Protein 8.7 g*

88. SESAME SOY CHICKEN SALAD

INGREDIENTS

- 150g of cooked chicken, shredded
- Large handful of chopped parsley (20g)
- ½ finely sliced red onion
- 60g of Pak choi, very finely shredded
- 100g of roughly chopped baby kale
- 1 peeled cucumber, slice in half lengthwise, remove seed and cut into slices
- 1 tablespoon of sesame seeds

For dressing:

- 2 teaspoons of soy sauce
- 1 teaspoon of clear honey
- Juice of 1 lime
- 1 teaspoon of sesame oil
- 1 tablespoon of extra virgin olive oil
- A few leaves, finely chopped oregano (skip this if using dried

DIRECTIONS

1. Clean your frying pan well and make sure it's dry, toast the sesame seeds for 2 minutes in the pan until fragrant and lightly browned. Set aside in a plate to cool.

To make the dressing:

2. Mix together the lime juice, soy sauce, olive oil, sesame oil and honey in a small bowl.
3. Place the kale, cucumber, parsley, red onion and Pak choi in a large bowl and mix gently. Pour dressing over salad and mix together.
4. Serve the salad in two different plates and add shredded chicken on top. Just before serving, sprinkle with sesame seeds.

Nutritions: *Kcal 304, Fat 6 g, Protein 33 g, Carbs 35 g*

89. SALMON CHICORY ROCKET SUPER SALAD

INGREDIENTS

- 10g of chopped lovage or celery leaves
- 10g of chopped parsley
- Juice ¼ lemon
- 1 tablespoon of extra-virgin olive oil
- 1 large medjool date, pitted and chopped
- 1 tablespoon of capers
- 15g of chopped walnuts
- 20g of sliced red onion
- 40g of sliced celery
- 80g of avocado, peeled, sliced
- 100g of smoked salmon slices or cooked chicken breast
- 50g of chicory leaves
- 50g of rocket

DIRECTIONS

1. On a large plate, place the salad leaves.
2. Mix together the remaining ingredients and spread mixture over leaves to serve.

Nutritions: *Kcal 300, Net carbs 30 g, Fat 21 g, Fiber 10 g, Protein 20 g*

90. FRESH CHOPPED SALAD WITH VINEGAR

INGREDIENTS

- 1/2 cup of fresh parsley, coarsely chopped
- 1/2 cup of Klamath olives, pitted and chopped coarsely
- Freshly ground pepper
- 4 medium seeded and diced tomatoes
- 2 tablespoons of white wine vinegar
- 1/2 cup of chopped scallions
- 1/2 teaspoon salt
- 2 cups of diced seedless cucumber
- 4 tablespoons of extra-virgin olive oil

DIRECTIONS

1. Add all the ingredients in a medium bowl; carefully toss to combine finely.
2. Serve after an hour.

Nutritions: *Kcal 113, Net carbs 5 g, Fat 10 g, Protein 1 g*

91. KING PRAWNS PARCELS

INGREDIENTS

- 2 lemon slices
- 50ml of vegetable stock
- 1 teaspoon of garlic crushed
- 300g of king prawns raw or cooked
- 2 thinly sliced broccoli florets
- 1 stick celery
- 1 courgette
- 1 carrot, peeled
- (Optional) Fresh dill

DIRECTIONS

1. Preheat your oven to 180°C or 160°C fans.
2. Shave the carrot, courgette and celery into ribbons with a veggie peeler and set aside.
3. Arrange two pieces of tin foil (large enough to hold your vegetables), add a smaller piece of grease-proof paper on top of each tin foil. Curl up edges so the filling can hold.
4. Add half of the vegetables over each piece of paper; add the prawns and a slice of lemon.
5. Mix vegetable stock with garlic and add on top the vegetables. Sprinkle top with dill if using. Seal the foil and transfer to the baking sheet.
6. Place the baking sheet in the oven and bake until vegetables are soft, about 10-15 minutes. Remove foil and serve.

Nutritions: *Kcal 204, Net carbs 4g, Fat 3g, Fiber 10g, Protein 36g*

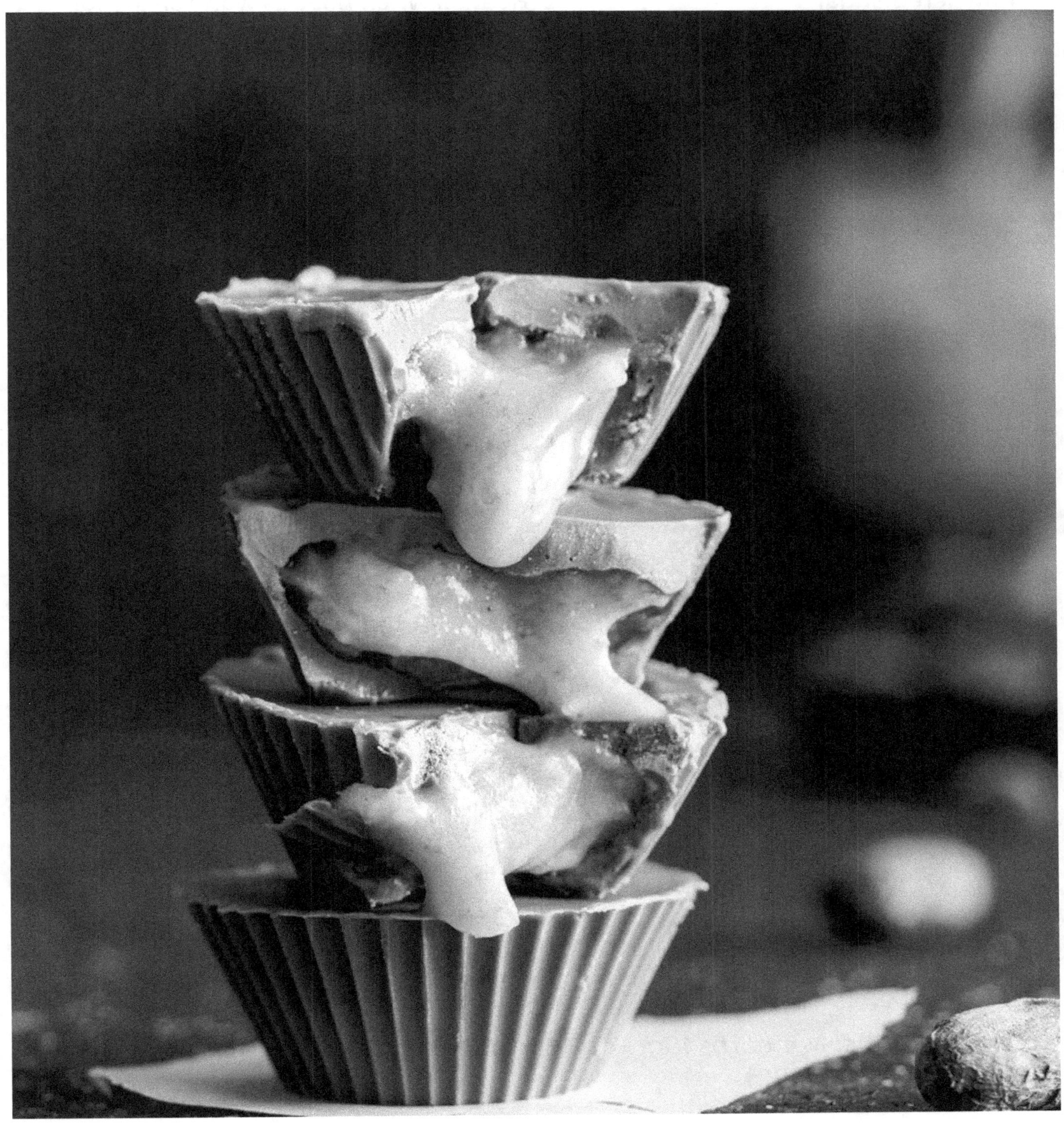

92. SNOW-FLAKES

INGREDIENTS

- Wonton wrappers
- Oil for frying
- Powdered-sugar

DIRECTIONS

1. Cut wonton wrappers just like you'd do a snowflake.
2. Heat oil when hot ads won-ton, fry for approximately 30 seconds, then reverse over.
3. Drain on a paper towel with powdered sugar.

Nutritions: *Net carbs 10g, Fat 3.69g, Fiber 3g, Protein 3g*

93. LEMON RICOTTA COOKIES WITH LEMON GLAZE

INGREDIENTS

- 2 1/2 cups all-purpose flour
- 1 teaspoon baking powder
- 1 teaspoon salt
- 1 tablespoon unsalted butter softened
- 2 cups sugar
- 2 capsules
- 1 teaspoon (15-ounce) container whole milk ricotta cheese
- 3 tablespoons lemon juice
- 1 lemon

Glaze:

- 11/2 cups powdered sugar
- 3 tbsps. Lemon juice
- 1 lemon

DIRECTIONS

1. Preheat the oven to 375°F.
2. In a medium bowl, combine the salt, flour, and baking powder. Set aside.
3. From the big bowl, blend the butter and the sugar levels. Get an electric mixer, beat the sugar and butter until light and fluffy, about three minutes. Add the eggs one at a time, beating until incorporated.
4. Insert the ricotta cheese, lemon juice and lemon zest. Beat to blend. Stir in the dry skin.
5. Line two baking sheets with parchment paper. Spoon the dough (approximately 2 tablespoons of each cookie) on the baking sheets. Bake for fifteen minutes, until slightly golden at the borders. Take out from the oven and leave the cookies— remaining the baking sheet for about 20 minutes.
6. Combine the powdered sugar, lemon juice and lemon peel in a small bowl and then stir until smooth. Spoon approximately ½ teaspoon on each cookie and make use of the back of the spoon to lightly disperse. Allow glaze harden for approximately two hours. Pack the biscuits in a decorative jar.

Nutritions: *Calories 123, Vitamin A and C, Protein 12 g*

94. HOMEMADE MARSHMALLOW FLUFF

INGREDIENTS

- 3/4 cups sugar
- 1/2 cup light corn syrup
- 1/4 cup water
- ⅛ teaspoon salt
- 3 little egg whites
- 1/4 teaspoon cream of tartar
- 1 teaspoon 1/2 teaspoon vanilla infusion

DIRECTIONS

1. In a little pan, mix together sugar, corn syrup, salt and water. Attach a candy thermometer into the side of this pan, which makes sure it will not touch the underside of the pan. Set aside.
2. From the bowl of a stand mixer, combine egg whites and cream of tartar. Begin to whip on medium speed with the whisk attachment.
3. Meanwhile, turn burner on top and place the pan with the sugar mix onto heat. Allow mix into a boil and heat to 240 degrees, stirring periodically.
4. The aim is to find the egg whites whipped to soft peaks and also the sugar heated to 240 degrees at near the same moment. Simply stop stirring the egg whites once they hit soft peaks.
5. Once the sugar has already reached 240 amounts, turn noodle onto reduce. Insert a little quantity of the popular sugar mix and let it mix. Insert still another little sum of the sugar mix. Carry on adding and mixing slowly, which means you never scramble the egg whites.
6. After all of the sugar was added into the egg whites, then turn the rate of this mixer and also keep overcoming concoction for around 79 minutes until the fluff remains glossy and stiff. In roughly the 5-minute mark, add vanilla extract.
7. Use the lint immediately or store it in an airtight container in the refrigerator.

Nutritions: *Kcal 534, Net carbs 40 g, Fat 35 g, Fiber 31 g, Protein 22 g*

95. GUILT TOTALLY FREE BANANA ICE-CREAM

INGREDIENTS

- 3 quite ripe bananas, peeled and rooted
- Couple of chocolate chips
- 2 tablespoons skim milk

DIRECTIONS

1. Put all the ingredients in a food processor and blend until creamy.
2. Eat freezes and appreciate afterward.

Nutritions: *Kcal 540, Net carbs 50 g, Fat 45 g, Fiber 17 g, Protein 15 g*

PREPARATION: 15 MIN   COOKING: 0 MIN   SERVES: 2

96. PERFECT LITTLE SNACK BALLS

INGREDIENTS

- 1/2 cup chunky peanut butter
- 3 tablespoons of flax seeds
- 3 tablespoons of wheat germ
- 1 tablespoon honey or agave
- 1/4 cup of powder

DIRECTIONS

1. Blend dry ingredients and adding from the honey and peanut butter.
2. Mix well and roll into chunks and then conclude by rolling into wheat germ.

Nutritions: *Kcal 200, Net carbs 30 g, Fat 28 g, Fiber 18 g, Protein 11 g*

97. DARK CHOCOLATE PRETZEL COOKIES

INGREDIENTS

- 1 cup yoghurt
- 1/2 teaspoon baking soda
- 1/4 teaspoon salt
- 1/4 teaspoon cinnamon
- 4 tablespoons butter softened
- 1/3 cup brown sugar
- 1 egg
- 1/2 teaspoon vanilla
- 1/2 cup dark chocolate chips
- 1/2 cup pretzels tsp. chopped

DIRECTIONS

1. Preheat oven to 350°F.
2. In a medium bowl, whisk together the sugar, butter, vanilla and egg.
3. In another bowl, stir together the flour, baking soda and salt.
4. Stir the bread mixture in using all the moist components, along with the chocolate chips and pretzels until just blended.
5. Drop large spoonful of dough on a baking tray without slope.
6. Bake 15-17 minutes, or until the bottom is crisp.
7. Allow to cool on a wire rack.

Nutritions: *Kcal 800, Net carbs 23 g, Fat 51 g, Fiber 32 g, Protein 43 g*

98. MASCARPONE CHEESECAKE WITH ALMOND CRUST

INGREDIENTS

Crust:

- 1/2 cup slivered almonds
- 8 teaspoons or 2/3 cups graham cracker crumbs
- 2 tablespoons sugar
- 1 tablespoon salted butter melted

Filling:

- 1 (8-ounce) package cream cheese, room temperature
- 1 (8-ounce) container mascarpone cheese, room temperature
- 3/4 cups sugar
- 1 teaspoon fresh lemon juice (or imitation lemon-juice)
- 1 teaspoon vanilla infusion
- 2 large eggs, room temperature

DIRECTIONS

For the crust:

1. Preheat oven to 350°F. Take per 9-inch diameter around the pan. Finely grind the almonds, cracker crumbs, sugar in a food processor. Bring the butter and process until moist crumbs form.
2. Press the almond mixture on the base of the prepared pan (maybe not on the surfaces of the pan). Bake the crust until it put and start to brown, about 1-2 minutes. Cool. Decrease the oven temperature to 325°F.

For your filling:

3. With an electric mixer, beat the cream cheese, mascarpone cheese, and sugar in a large bowl until smooth, occasionally scraping down the sides of the jar using a rubber spatula. Beat in the lemon juice and vanilla. Add the eggs, one at a time, beating until combined after each addition.
4. Pour the cheese mixture on the crust from the pan. Put the pan into a big skillet or Pyrex dish, pour enough hot water to the roasting pan to come halfway up the sides of one's skillet. Bake until the middle of this racket goes slightly when the pan is gently shaken, about 1 hour (the dessert will get business if it's cold). Transfer the cake to a stand; trendy for 1 hour. Refrigerate until the cheesecake is cold, at least eight hours.
5. Topping squeezed just a small thick cream in the microwave using a busted up chocolate brown—afterward, get a plastic bag and cut out a hole at the corner—then pour the melted chocolate to the baggie and use this to decorate the cake!

Nutritions: *Kcal 534, Net carbs 18 g, Fat 22 g, Fiber 17 g, Protein 32 g*

99. MARSHMALLOW POPCORN BALLS

INGREDIENTS

- 2 bags microwave popcorn
- 1 12.6 ounce tote M&M's
- 3 cups honey roasted peanuts
- 1 package 16 ounce massive marshmallows
- 1 cup butter, cubed

DIRECTIONS

1. In a bowl, blend the popcorn, peanuts and M&M's.
2. In a big pot, combine marshmallows and butter.
3. Cook medium-low warmth.
4. Insert popcorn mix, blend nicely
5. Spray muffin tins with nonstop cooking spray.
6. When cool enough to handle, spray hands together with non-stick cooking spray and then shape into chunks and put into the muffin tin to carry contour.
7. Add Popsicle stick into each chunk and then let cool.
8. Wrap each person in vinyl when chilled.

Nutritions: *Kcal 300, Net carbs 24 g, Fat 23 g, Fiber 34 g, Protein 30 g*

100. HOMEMADE ICE-CREAM DRUMSTICKS

INGREDIENTS

- Vanilla ice cream
- 2 hazelnut chunks
- Magical shell of chocolate
- Sugar levels
- Nuts
- Parchment newspaper

DIRECTIONS

1. Soften the ice cream and mix the topping (two sliced hazel nut balls).
2. Fill underside of sugar with magic and nut shells and top with ice-cream.
3. Wrap parchment paper round cone and then fill cone over about 1.5 inches across the cap of the cone (the newspaper can help to carry its shape).
4. Shirt with magical nuts and shells.
5. Freeze for about 20 minutes, before ice-cream is business.

Nutritions: *Kcal 546, Net carbs 25 g, Fat 20 g, Fiber 21 g, Protein 18 g*

101. ULTIMATE CHOCOLATE CHIP COOKIE FUDGE BROWNIE BAR

INGREDIENTS

- 1 cup (2 sticks) butter, softened
- 1 cup granulated sugar
- 3/4 cup light brown sugar
- 2 big eggs
- 1 tablespoon pure vanilla extract
- 2 1/2 cups all-purpose flour
- 1 teaspoon baking soda
- 1 teaspoon lemon
- 2 cups (12 ounces) milk chocolate chips
- Inch per kg double stuffed Oreos
- Inch family-size (9×1-3) brownie mixture
- 1/4 cup hot fudge topping

DIRECTIONS

1. Preheat oven to 350°F.
2. Mix the butter and sugars in a large bowl, using an electric mixer at medium speed for 35 minutes.
3. Add the vanilla and eggs and mix well to thoroughly combine. In another bowl, whisk together the flour, baking soda and salt, and slowly incorporate in the mixer till the bread is simply combined.
4. Stir in chocolate chips.
5. Spread the cookie dough at the bottom of a 9×1-3 baking dish that is wrapped with wax paper and then coated with cooking spray.
6. Shirt with a coating of Oreos. Mix together brownie mix, adding an optional 1/4 cup of hot fudge directly into the mixture.
7. Twist the brownie batter within the cookie-dough and Oreos.
8. Cover with foil and bake at 350°F for half an hour.
9. Remove foil and continue baking for another 15-25 minutes. Let cool before cutting on brownies might nevertheless be gooey at the midst while warm, but will also place up perfectly once chilled.

Nutritions: *Kcal 490, Net carbs 29 g, Fat 27 g, Fiber 16 g, Protein 32 g*

102. CRUNCHY CHOCOLATE CHIP COCONUT MACADAMIA NUT COOKIES

INGREDIENTS

- 1 cup yogurt
- 1/2 teaspoon baking soda
- 1/2 teaspoon salt
- 1 tablespoon of butter, softened
- 1 cup firmly packed brown sugar
- 1/2 cup sugar
- 1 big egg
- 1/2 cup semi-sweet chocolate chips
- 1/2 cup sweet coconut flakes
- 1/2 cup coarsely chopped roasted walnuts macadamia nuts
- 1/2 cup raisins

DIRECTIONS

1. Preheat the oven to 325°f.
2. In a little bowl, whisk together the flour, oats and baking soda and salt; then place a side.
3. In your mixer bowl, mix together the butter/sugar/egg mix.
4. Mix from the flour/oats mix until just combined and stir in the chocolate chips, raisins, nuts and coconut.
5. Decked outsized bits on a parchment-lined cookie sheet.
6. Bake for 1-3 minutes before biscuits are only barely golden brown.
7. Remove from the oven and then leave the cookie sheets to cool at least 10 minutes.

Nutritions: *Kcal 657, Net carbs 20 g, Fat 45 g, Fiber 54 g, Protein 32 g*

103. PIZZA KALE CHIPS

INGREDIENTS

- 1 teaspoon dried oregano
- 1 teaspoon dried marjoram
- 1 teaspoon garlic powder
- 1 teaspoon onion powder
- 8 cups kale leaves from about six stalks, veins removed
- 1 cup raw cashews
- 1/2 cup tomato paste, one small can
- 2 tablespoons Nutritional Yeast, Lewis Labs Brewer's Yeast Buds (from sugar beets)
- 1/2 teaspoon salt
- 1/4 teaspoon red pepper flakes
- 1 teaspoon dried basil
- 1/2 teaspoon dried rosemary

DIRECTIONS

1. Place the cashews in a tub, cover with filtered water and allow the cashews, preferably overnight, to soak refrigerated for at least 2 hours.
2. Drain away the cashew juice. Place the cashews in a meal processor or blender. To only cover the cashews, apply filtered water, and heat until creamy smooth.
3. Stir together the cashew cream in a large mixing bowl with all remaining ingredients except the kale. Stir until the combination is even.
4. Rinse the kale and take the leaves off the fibrous roots. Tear the pieces into "chip" size.
5. Take the kale away with the cashew cream filled with "pizza." You may need to do this a little bit at a time, making sure that coverage is assured.
6. Dehydrate the kale chips for 12 hours, and then cook at 105-115 degrees.

Nutritions: *Kcal 345, Net carbs 470 g, Fat 50 g, Fiber 19 g, Protein 32 g*

104. BAKED POTATOES WITH SPICY CHICKPEA STEW

INGREDIENTS

- 4-6 baking potatoes, pricked all over
- 2 tablespoons olive oil
- 4 cloves garlic, grated or crushed
- 2cm ginger, grated
- 2 red onions, finely chopped
- ½ - 2 teaspoons chili flakes
- 2 tablespoons cumin seeds
- 2 tablespoons turmeric
- Splash of water
- 2 x 14-ounce tins chopped tomatoes
- 2 tablespoons unsweetened cocoa powder (or cacao)
- 2 x 14-ounce tin chickpeas (or kidney beans if you prefer), including the chickpea water. Don't drain!!
- 2 yellow peppers (or the color you prefer), chopped into bite size pieces
- 2 tablespoons parsley, plus extra for garnish
- Salt and pepper to taste (optional)
- Side salad (optional)

DIRECTIONS

1. Preheat the oven to 200°C while you can prepare all the supplies you need.
2. Put your baking potatoes in the oven when the oven is hot enough, and cook them for 1 hour or until they are done as you like them.
3. Place the olive oil and chopped red onion in a large, wide saucepan once the potatoes are in the oven and cook gently with the lid until the onions are soft but not brown for 5 minutes.
4. Remove the lid and add the garlic, cumin, ginger, and chili. Cook on low heat for another minute, then add the turmeric and a really slight splash of water and cook for another minute, taking care not to let the saucepan get too hot.
5. Add cocoa powder, chickpeas (including chickpea water), and yellow pepper on the tomatoes. Put to boil and cook for 45 minutes at low heat until the sauce is heavy and unctuous (but don't let it burn!). The stew should be handled at the same time as the potatoes.
6. At last, stir in the two tablespoons of parsley and some salt and pepper, if desired, and serve the stew over the baked potatoes, perhaps with a simple side salad.

Nutritions: *Kcal 200, Net carbs 240 g, Fat 34 g, Fiber 16 g, Protein 20 g*

105. APRICOT OATMEAL COOKIES

INGREDIENTS

- 1/2 cup (1 stick) butter, softened
- 2/3 cups light brown sugar packed
- Inch egg
- 3/4 cups all-purpose flour
- 1/2 teaspoon baking soda
- 1/2 teaspoon vanilla infusion
- 1/2 teaspoon cinnamon
- 1/4 teaspoon salt
- 1 teaspoon 1/2 cups chopped oats
- 3/4 cups yolks
- 1/4 cup sliced apricots
- 1/3 cup slivered almonds

DIRECTIONS

1. Preheat oven to 350°F.
2. In a big bowl, combine with the butter, sugar and egg until smooth.
3. In another bowl, whisk the flour, baking soda, cinnamon and salt together.
4. Stir the dry ingredients to the butter-sugar bowl.
5. Now stir in the oats, raisins, apricots and almonds.

Nutritions: *Kcal 650, Net carbs 25 g, Fat 20 g, Fiber 15 g, Protein 22 g*

106. CREPES LEEKS AND MUSHROOMS

INGREDIENTS

- 80g white flour
- 20g of chickpea flour
- 200ml of soy milk
- 100g of sliced and cooked champignon mushrooms
- 2 leeks (including the pale green part)
- Soya cream
- Chives
- Garlic powder

DIRECTIONS

1. First mix the two flours in a bowl, then add the milk a little at a time, stirring with a whisk to avoid the formation of lumps. As much as you want, salt the dough.
2. Fry the thinly sliced leeks in a frying pan. When they are tender, add the mushrooms and stir for a few minutes. Add a little soy cream, let it set aside.
3. In the meantime, prepare the crepes: oil a non-stick pan for crepes with the special brush and pour half the mixture, taking care to cover the entire surface of the pan in a thin layer. Let the other side cozy up, turn and cook too. Stuff it with half the stuffing and roll it up. Repeat the operation for the second crêpe.
4. In a small bowl, mix soy cream with salt, pepper, chives and garlic powder. Pour the sauce over the pancakes when serving.

Notes:

It is better to use the champignons already cooked because of cooking them together with the leeks you lose the taste of the latter.

Nutritions: *Kcal 450, Net carbs 30 g, Fat 15 g, Fiber 21 g, Protein 13 g*

107. EGGPLANT CROQUETTES

INGREDIENTS

- 2 round Aubergine (about 600g)
- 1 slice of stale bread
- Unsweetened soy milk
- 1 tablespoon of yeast
- 2 tablespoons of chickpea flour
- 2 tablespoons of flour
- Parsley
- Bread crumbs
- Frying oil

DIRECTIONS

1. Wash the eggplants, pierce with a fork and let them wither in the oven for about 20 minutes.
2. Make them cool, cut them in half and with a spoon extract the pulp and put it in a bowl; add the slice of bread softened in milk and well squeezed, chopped parsley, yeast and flour, salt and mix.
3. Form oval croquettes, pass them in breadcrumbs and fry them in hot oil.

Nutritions: *Kcal 350, Net carbs 18 g, Fat 22 g, Fiber 13 g, Protein 6 g*

108. ZUCCHINI CROQUETTES

INGREDIENTS

- 500g zucchini
- 2 slices of bread box
- 2 tablespoons of yeast
- 2 tablespoons of bread crumbs
- 4 tablespoons of oat flakes
- Half a glass of soya milk
- Nutmeg

DIRECTIONS

1. Wash the zucchini, trim them and scratch them with the vegetable grater; dip the slices of bread in soy milk, heat over very low heat, squeeze them and add them to the zucchini.
2. Add the baking powder, bread crumbs, oatmeal flakes, nutmeg and salt. Mix well, form croquettes with wet hands, compact them well and fry in hot oil. Drain and serve hot.
3. Raw zucchini tends to purge water, so if the mixture is too moist, increase the quantity of oat flakes, otherwise these very delicate croquettes could flake during cooking.

Nutritions: *Kcal 450, Net carbs 24 g, Fat 35 g, Fiber 18 g, Protein 23 g*

109. DOMES

INGREDIENTS

- 1 roll of vegan puff pastry
- Frozen peas
- Frozen mushrooms
- Soya cream
- Oil
- Garlic

DIRECTIONS

1. Fold the puff pastry, cut the circles (about 12cm in diameter) with the help of a cup. Brush dough circles with water and form into foil, place in the oven at 160°C for 10 minutes, cover with foil, and bake for another 10 minutes. Meanwhile, prepare the filling by frying the peas and mushrooms separately in a little oil and half a clove of garlic.
2. Remove the domes from the oven, gently remove them from the forms and fill them with peas and mushrooms, mixed with a few tablespoons of soya cream. Before serving, put the domes back in the oven to enhance the crunchiness of the puff pastry.

Notes:

The filling can vary: instead of cream you can use béchamel sauce, as fillings are suitable spinach and vegan ricotta cheese, slices of soya sausage with pieces of mozzarella... and everything the imagination suggests.

Nutritions: *Kcal 600, Net carbs 34 g, Fat 30 g, Fiber 9 g, Protein 19 g*

110. DICED SEITAN AND LENTILS

INGREDIENTS

- 4 slices of seitan
- 1 box of lentils
- Half onion
- 1 tablespoon of soy cream
- Salt and pepper
- A tablespoon of extra virgin olive oil
- A handful of fresh parsley
- Turmeric (optional)

DIRECTIONS

1. Cut the seitan into cubes. Cut the onion and fry it in oil. When it is well colored—but not burnt—add the seitan cubes and, after a few minutes, the lentils drained and well washed. Add salt and pepper and sauté with a little hot water. Finish with the cream, turmeric and chopped parsley, cook a few more minutes and then serve with a nice fresh salad and toasted whole meal bread.

Nutritions: *Kcal 333, Net carbs 10 g, Fat 33 g, Fiber 15 g, Protein 11 g*

111. DICED TOFU AND LENTILS

INGREDIENTS

- 200g of tofu cake
- Soy sauce (shoyu)
- Extra virgin olive oil
- An onion
- A sprig of rosemary
- 2 tablespoons of chopped chili pepper
- 50g of red lentils
- Vegetable stock
- Bread crumbs

DIRECTIONS

1. Marinate the diced tofu for half an hour in the soy sauce, adding a little water to cover it. In the meantime, boil the red lentils, previously washed, in the vegetable stock for about 20 minutes, until they are soft enough and the stock has dried a bit.
2. Then sauté 2 tablespoons of chili pepper, the diced onion and rosemary in olive oil until the onion is golden brown and the sauté takes on the smell of spices. Add the tofu with some of the marinating shoyu and after a few minutes also the lentils with very little broth.
3. Let everything shrink with the lid and over low heat and to thicken, add 2 tablespoons of bread crumbs.

Notes

I accompanied the dish with a side dish of boiled green beans and soy sprouts covered with mustard sauce previously diluted with soy milk.

Nutritions: *Kcal 543, Net carbs 16 g, Fat 33 g, Fiber 12 g, Protein 6 g*

21-DAY MEAL PLAN

DAY	BREAKFAST	LUNCH	DINNER	SNACKS/ DESSERTS
1	Kale & Orange Juice	Cinnamon Buckwheat Bowls	Bang-bang Chicken Noodle	Walnuts Avocado Salad
2	Matcha Green Juice	Sirtfood Salmon Salad	Full-of-veg Hash	Poached Pear Salad With Dijon Vinegar Dressing
3	Celery Juice	Broccoli Salad	Cajun steak and Veg Rice Jar	Snow-Flakes
4	Pancakes with Apples and Blackcurrants	Fresh Herb Frittata	Sri Lankan-Style Sweet Potato Curry	Lemon Ricotta Cookies With Lemon Glaze
5	Chocolate Waffles	Arugula, Egg, and Charred Asparagus Salad	Pesto Salmon Pasta Noodles	Homemade Marshmallow Fluff
6	Salmon & Kale Omelet	Spring Vegetable and Quinoa Salad with Bacon	Chicken Liver along with Tomato Ragu	Guilt Totally Free Banana Ice-cream

7	Black Forest Smoothie	Golden Chicory in Prosciutto Wraps	Minted Lamb with a Couscous Salad	Perfect Little Snack Balls
8	Savory Turmeric Pancakes with Lemon Yogurt Sauce	Vegetable Cabbage Soup	Jack Fruit Tortilla Bowls	Dark chocolate Pizza Kale Chips
9	Kale and Blackcurrant Smoothie	Fresh Herb Frittata	Carrot, Courgette and Halloumi Hamburgers	Apricot Oatmeal Cookies
10	Apple & Cucumber Juice	Herb-Roasted Olives and Tomatoes	Rita's 'Rowdy' enchiladas	Mascarpone Cheesecake with Almond Crust
11	Kale & Raspberry Salad	Grilled Asparagus with Caper Vinaigrette	Bacon and egg fried rice	Marshmallow Popcorn Balls
12	Buckwheat Pancakes	Herby Pork with Apple & Chicory Salad	Super-speedy Prawn Risotto	Homemade Ice-Cream Drumsticks
13	Arugula & Berries Salad	Chia, Quinoa & Avocado Salad	Miso Marinated Cod with Stir-Fried Greens and Sesame	Ultimate Chocolate Chip Cookie Fudge Brownie Bar
14	Kale & Citrus Fruit Salad	Tomato Green Bean Soup	Bulgur Appetizer Salad	Crunchy Chocolate Chip Coconut Macadamia Nut Cookies

15	Vegetable & Nut Loaf	Kale Salad with Pecorino and Lemon	Cocoa Bars	Pizza Kale Chips
16	Kale Scramble	Cinnamon Buckwheat Bowls	Cinnamon Apple Chips	Diced Seitan And Lentils
17	Kale & Citrus Fruit Salad	Grilled Asparagus with Caper Vinaigrette	Greek Party Dip	Apricot Oatmeal Cookies
18	Dates & Parma Ham	Herb-Roasted Olives and Tomatoes	Spicy Pumpkin Seeds Bowls	Crepes Leeks and Mushrooms
19	Scrambled Eggs with Mushrooms	Fresh Herb Frittata	Apple and Pecans Bowls	Eggplant Croquettes
20	Blueberry Muffins	Golden Chicory in Prosciutto Wraps	Shrimp Muffins	Zucchini Croquettes
21	Pink Omelets	Broccoli Salad	Zucchini Bowls	Diced Seitan And Lentils

BUILDING A DIET
THAT WORKS

We were doing something different with the Sirtfood Diet. We took the strongest Sirtfoods on the planet and woven them in a brand-new way of eating, the likes of which were never seen before. We picked the "best of the best" from the healthiest diets, we have ever seen and built a world-beating diet from them.

The good news is; you don't immediately have to follow an Okinawan's traditional diet or eat like an Italian mamma, on the Sirtfood Diet is not only utterly unrealistic but unnecessary. Sure, one thing you might be taken by from the Sirtfoods list is their familiarity. Although you may not consume all the items on the menu at the moment, you are most definitely eating others. Then why didn't you just lose weight already?

The answer is found as we explore the various elements that the most cutting-edge nutrition science indicates are needed to build a workable diet. It is about eating the right amount of Sirtfoods, range, and shape. It's about applying ample protein portions to the Sirtfood plates, and then enjoying your meals at the best time of day. And it's about the right to consume the authentic, savory things you love in the amounts you want.

Hitting Your Quota

Most people just don't eat nearly enough Sirtfoods right now to evoke a strong fat-burning and health-boosting effect. Once researchers looked at the use of five primary nutrient-activating sirtuins (quercetin, myricetin, kaempferol, lute Olin, and apigenin) in the US diet, human dietary intakes were found to be miserably 13 milligrams a day. Conversely, the average Japanese consumption was five times greater. Compare this with our Sirtfood Diet experiment, where everyday individuals ate hundreds of milligrams of sirtuin-activating nutrients.

What we are thinking about is a true diet change in which we raise by as much as fifty times our daily intake of sirtuin-activating nutrients. While that may sound overwhelming or unrealistic, it isn't really. Through taking all our top Sirtfoods and bringing them together in a way that is fully compatible with your busy life, you too can quickly and effectively reach the level of consumption required to enjoy all of the benefits.

Heard a Term 'Synergy'?

We believe it's better to eat a wide range of these wonder nutrients in the form of natural whole grains, where they coexist with the hundreds of other bio-active plant chemicals that act synergistically to improve our wellbeing. We think working for a design is more comfortable, rather than against it. It is for this purpose that single nutrient supplements fail to show time and time again.

Take, for example, the classic nutrient resveratrol, which activates sirtuin. In supplement form, it is poorly absorbed; but in its natural food matrix of red wine, its bio-availability (how much the body can use) is at least six times higher. Add to this the fact that red wine produces not only one, but a whole host of sirtuin activating polyphenols that function together to offer health benefits, including piceatannol, quercetin, myricetin, and epicatechin. Or we could turn our attention from the turmeric to curcumin.

Curcumin is well established to be the critical sirtuin-activating nutrient in turmeric. Yet, research shows that whole turmeric has better PPAR-y activity for fighting fat loss and is more effective at inhibiting cancer and reducing blood sugar levels than curcumin in isolation. It's not hard to see why isolating a single element in its entire food process is nowhere near as effective as eating it.

But what makes a dietary strategy different is when we start mixing several Sirtfoods. For starters, we are further enhancing the bio-availability of resveratrol-containing foods by bringing in quercetin-rich Sirtfoods. Not only this, but they complement each other with their acts. Both are fat busters, but there are variations of how each of them is doing this. Resveratrol is beneficial in helping to kill current fat cells, while quercetin excels in avoiding the formation of new fat cells. In addition, all sides target fat, resulting in a more significant impact on the reduction of weight than just eating large amounts of a single food.

And this is a trend which we see again and again. Foods rich in sirtuin activator apigenin improve quercetin absorption from food and enhance its function. Quercetin, in effect, is synergistic with epigallocatechin gallate (EGCG) behavior. Yet EGCG's service with curcumin is synergistic. And so, it begins. Not only are specific whole foods more effective than single ingredients, but we tap into an entire tapestry of health benefits that nature has weaved—so intricate, so pure, it's impossible to try to beat it.

Juices and Food

Sirtfood Diet is a portion of both juices and whole foods. Here we are thinking about juices explicitly made from a juicer—blenders and smoothie makers (such as the NutriBullet) will not work. For many, this will seem counter-intuitive, based on the fact that the fiber is lost when something is juiced. But this is just what we want for leafy greens.

Feed fiber includes what is called non-extractable polyphenols (or NEPPs). These are polyphenols, called sirtuin activators, which are bound to the fibrous portion of the food and only activated by our pleasant gut bacteria until broken down. We don't get the NEPPs by cutting the yarn, so miss out on their beauty. Importantly, though, the NEPP content varies dramatically based on the plant size. The NEPP quality in foods such as meat, cereals, and nuts are substantial and should be consumed whole (NEPPs contain over 50 percent of polyphenols in strawberries!). But for leafy vegetables, the active ingredients in the Sirtfood drink, they are much lower despite having a significant fiber content.

So, when it comes to leafy greens, by juicing them and eliminating the low-nutrient fiber we get full bang for our buck, so we can use even larger volumes and obtain a super concentrated hit of sirtuin-activating polyphenols.

There's another benefit of cutting the thread, too. Leafy greens comprise a form of fiber called insoluble fiber, which has a digestive scrubbing effect. But when we take too much of it, it can irritate and hurt our gut lining just like if we over-scrub stuff. This suggests that for many individuals, leafy green-packed smoothies can overwhelm fiber, possibly aggravating or even inducing IBS (irritable bowel syndrome) and hampering our nutrient absorption.

So, the bottom line is that we need to develop a lifestyle that blends all beverages and whole foods for maximum benefit to get the sirtuin genes going for dramatic weight loss and wellness.

Power of Protein

Its plants bring the Sirt into the Sirtfood Diet. However, Sirtfood meals should always be rich in protein to gain maximum benefit. It has been shown that a building block of the dietary protein named leucine has additional benefits in activating SIRT to enhance fat burning and boost blood sugar control.

But leucine also has another part, and this is where it shines through its synergistic partnership with Sirtfoods. Leucine effectively induces anabolism (building things) in our cells, particularly in the muscle, which requires a great deal of energy and ensures that our energy factories (called mitochondria) have to work overtime. It induces a need for the Sirtfoods operation inside our cells. As you may remember, one of the effects of Sirtfoods is to promote the development of more mitochondria, to increase their performance, and to allow them to burn fat as fuel. Our bodies, then need these to satisfy this extra demand for energy. The upshot is that we see a synergistic effect when mixing Sirtfoods with dietary protein that enhances sirtuin activation and ultimately gets you to burn fat to support muscle growth and better safety. For this purpose, the meals in the book are built to provide a large protein portion.

Oily fish is an exceptionally good protein alternative to supplement Sirtfoods' action because they are high in omega-3 fatty acids alongside their protein content. There is no way that you will have read a lot about the health benefits of oily fish and especially omega-3 fish oils. And now, recent research suggests that the advantages of omega-3 fats that come from enhancing the functioning of our sirtuin genes.

Over the past few years, many concerns have been raised about the adverse effects of protein-rich diets on wellbeing, and without Sirtfoods to counterbalance the protein, we can start to understand why. Leucine can be a knife with two-edges. We need Sirtfoods, as we have seen, to help our cells fulfill the metabolic demand that leucine imposes upon them. Without them, though, our mitochondria can become unstable, so high levels of leucine will promote obesity and insulin resistance, rather than improve health. Sirtfoods help not only hold the symptoms of leucine in check but also function effectively in our favor.

Speak of leucine as putting the foot on the weight loss and wellness generator, with Sirtfoods, the tool that ensures that the cell satisfies the increased demand. The engine blows, without the Sirtfoods.

Returning to questions about the health effects of protein-rich diets, the missing piece of the puzzle is Sirtfoods. Usually, the US diet is protein-rich but requires Sirtfoods to counterbalance it, which makes it essential for Sirtfoods to become an integral part of how Americans live.

Try to Eat Early

The theory is the sooner, the better when it comes to food, preferably done feeding for the day by 7 p.m. for two significant reasons. Firstly, to harvest the Sirtfoods natural satiating power. Eating a meal that will leave you feeling full, happy, and energized as you go about your day is much more useful than spending the entire day exploring hungry just to feed and remain full while you sleep through the night.

But there's a second good reason to keep eating habits in line with your inner body clock. We also have an internal biological clock, called our circadian rhythm, which controls all of our normal body functions according to daytime.

This affects, among other things, how the body handles the food we eat. Our clocks operate in synchrony, above all observing the signals of the sun's light-dark cycle. We're programmed as a diurnal species to be busy in the daytime rather than at night.

The body clock, then allows us to handle food more efficiently during the day when it's bright, and we're supposed to be busy, and less so when it's night, where we're primed for rest and sleep instead.

The question is that many of us have "work clocks" and "social clocks," which are not aligned with the sun's slowing down. Sometimes after dark is the only option; some of us get to sleep. At some point, we will teach our body clock in synchronizing with different schedules, including "evening Chrono types" that want or need to be busy, eat and sleep later in the day. Life misaligned from the light-dark environmental process, therefore, comes at a cost.

PERSONAL
SIRT JOURNEY

One more month, another popular diet fanning out quickly over the web.

The most recent eating fever is known as the Sirtfood Diet, and it's grabbing individuals' eye for a couple of reasons. One, it lets you eat stuff like chocolate. Two, it guarantees enormous outcomes immediately—seven pounds in seven days. Also, three, it includes eating "sirtfoods," a mysterious gathering of nourishments that, as far as anyone knows, contain incredible fat-consuming mixes.

These elements have helped the Sirtfood Diet get on large in England, and it's beginning to advance over the lake. In any case, is the Sirtfood Diet truly a decent method to eat more beneficial? Or, on the other hand, is it merely one more prevailing fashion of-the-month diet destined to be overlooked?

What are Sirtfoods?

The front of The Sirtfood Diet book calls them "wonder nourishments that turbo-charge weight loss," yet that seems like an impervious promoting language. So, what precisely are these marvel nourishments?

Sirtuins (abbreviation for Silent Information Regulars) are a class of normally happening proteins in the human body. First found a couple of decades prior, they have energizing capacities, inquire about shows. The exploration contemplates never performed on genuine individuals (selecting instead of test cylinders or lab creatures). However, sirtuins have been found to assume a job in clearing free radicals, lessening irritation, managing our inner clock, and forestalling maturing. The exploration has persuaded that sirtuins might be utilized to treat or forestall certain infections, like malignant growth and Type 2 Diabetes.

It's additionally been discovered that sirtuins might keep fat cells from copying. The proof isn't firm, yet this is the place the "turbo-charge weight loss" guarantee of the Sirtfood Diet originates from.

Sirtfoods are nourishments strong in sirtuin activators. Sirtuin activators transmit messages to our DNA to expand the creation of sirtuin proteins. In principle, eating more sirtfoods brings about a more noteworthy creation of sirtuin proteins and every one of the advantages they bring. This is the essential reason for the Sirtfood Diet—eat more extra sirtfoods, provide more sirtuins, and get more fit, decrease aggravation, live more, and so on.

The Diet Plan

The nourishments prescribed by the diet incorporate dull chocolate, blueberries, espresso, arugula, kale, buckwheat, green tea, parsley, additional virgin olive oil, pecans, onions, turmeric and that's just the beginning.

During the initial three days of the diet, you drink two green squeezes and eat only one dinner every day. During this time, you are restricted to 1,000 calories each day. Throughout the following four days, you take two juices for each day and consume two dinners every day, while constraining yourself to 1,500 calories for each day. After the principal week and for the following 14 days, you expend an abundance of sirtfoods in three dinners and one juice for every day. Following 21 days, the center changes to "Sirtifying" your preferred suppers by embedding's or subbing sirtfoods into plans.

Obviously, the advantages of the Sirtfood Diet come rather rapidly. Numerous dieters report significant weight loss and expanded vitality in the simpler days.

The Analysis

One clear warning with the Sirtfood Diet is its guarantee of large outcomes in a brief timeframe.

The book has a major red sticker on the spread, yelling that members will "lose 7 lbs. in 7 days." These kinds of cases regularly demonstrate diets looking to sucker individuals who are edgy to shed pounds, not diets planned for helping individuals make durable lifestyle changes. The "convenient solution" guarantee sets unreasonable desires for dieters, who may be persuaded they can keep on getting in shape at that emotional rate past multi-week. Genuine, manageable weight loss is generally accomplished by shedding a couple of pounds seven days. "I wouldn't be a major aficionado of supporting this kind of eating where it centers on losing a great deal of weight in a short measure of time," says enlisted dietitian Travis Piattoly, who works as a sustenance advisor to the New Orleans Saints and New Orleans Pelicans. "A great deal of the weight will be water and potentially even muscle tissue."

Additionally, the calorie limitations during the principal week could be out and out risky, particularly if you're a competitor or dynamic individual. Competitors live exceptionally dynamic lifestyles, and young people need a greater number of calories than grown-ups significantly to help legitimate development. Albeit a calorie shortage is the way to getting thinner, too enormous a deficiency can cause issues like constant weariness and absence of core interest. NFL All-Pro guarded end J. J. Watt as of late felt the depleting impacts of a huge calorie shortfall and had to make some genuine diet changes to remain sharp.

Past the principal week, the center shifts from calorie-including to eating dinners high in sirtfoods. This is commonly a nice thought since most of the nourishments associated with the

Sirtfood Diet are profoundly nutritious. They're plant-based nourishments, low in calories and high in fiber, protein, nutrients, cancer prevention agents, and phytochemicals. They're additionally substantially more difficult to gorge than profoundly handled nourishments.

Nonetheless, the entire "sirtuin activator" thing most likely assumes to a lesser extent a job in the intensity of sirtfoods than the remainder of their nourishing profile. Berries and kale are routes preferred for you over treats and chips, whether or not they contain sirtuin activators. If you begin eating more plant-based nourishments, you're going to feel much improved— it's actually that basic.

The Verdict

We praise the Sirtfood Diet for its emphasis on eating more plant-based nourishments; however, it's unquestionably not an ideal diet.

The underlying calorie limitations are unreasonably exacting for some individuals, and the guarantee of seven pounds of weight loss in the initial seven days is anything but a solid methodology. The huge spotlight on sirtuins is likewise somewhat odd since the exploration of sirtuins (and specifically, their job in weight the executives) is as yet starter. The sirtfoods remembered for the Sirtfood Diet are, for the most part, sound plant-based nourishments high in an assortment of supplements. We're speculating a great many different supplements and mixes in these nourishments (the majority of which are well-examined than sirtuin activators) are the genuine motivation behind why individuals are revealing sirtfoods assist them with feeling and look better. A lot of sound nourishments are excluded from the Sirtfood Diet and maintaining a strategic distance from them exclusively, considering that it is absolutely superfluous.

If you're hoping to get more fit, your initial step ought to be to eliminate refined sugar items (pop, treats, and so on) and excursions to the drive-through. Supplant those nourishments with plant-based alternatives and drink more water. If you're eating the correct sorts of nourishments, the amount you're eating shouldn't be a significant issue.

You should likewise meet with a wellbeing proficient or enlisted dietitian. They can customize an arrangement for you as opposed to utilizing the "one-size-fits-all" approach numerous trend diets depend on. What's more, recollect—gradual advancement is often the most secure and the most manageable approach to getting more fit.

The Sirtfood Diet: the most recent in a not insignificant rundown of BS faddy diets customers, companions, and family, have sent me for my expert scrutinize. I figured that if they were asking, then others must have questions as well. This is a quite extensive book, so here's the TL: DR - this diet is false, don't get the book, and work with a qualified nutritionist.

Still With Me? How About We Separate It

Most importantly, we have to comprehend what sirtfoods are and to get that, and we have to realize what sirtuins are. You all prepared for a little science? Here we go.

Sirtuins are a gathering of proteins known as SIRs. They were found in people a couple of decades prior and have been forcefully examined from that point forward, for the most part, at a subcellular level or in lab creatures (for example, very few examinations on genuine human individuals). This has driven researchers to make energizing disclosures about the job of these proteins in securing metabolic wellbeing, including guideline of our natural tickers (otherwise known as circadian cadence), lessening irritation, wiping up free radicals that can make harm DNA, assisting with ensuring the honesty of our DNA and keep it from untimely maturing; therefore, SIRs may assume a significant job in counteraction of Alzheimer's. Researchers likewise figure they might be significant in securing against (and perhaps treating) illnesses like sort two diabetes, cardiovascular sicknesses like respiratory failures and stroke, and even a few tumors. Really energizing stuff, isn't that so? Right! Be that as it may, it's imperative to state that, although these discoveries are promising, they're: 1) reductionist in nature (for example, we don't simply eat just sirtfoods) and 2) we don't have numerous examinations in people yet.

Anyway, sirtuins have been embroiled in keeping fat cells from copying; a wonder is known as abiogenesis (fat cells being the Latin for fat) (just kidding, yet fat means fat). It was now that the creators of 'The Sirtfood Diet' heard a 'KA-CHING' and saw little $ drifting before them.

Along these lines, the hypothesis is then, that specific nourishments can up-regulate the declaration of the SIR qualities. Every one of that implies is that sure nourishments send messages to our DNA to instruct them to make a greater amount of the sirtuin proteins. In this way, more sirtfoods = more sirt proteins. Alright? It's somewhat more muddled than that, yet you get the thought.

The creators of TSD made this a stride further and essentially arrived at the resolution that if you make a diet up of a lot of these alleged 'sirtfoods' you'll not just impact individuals' fat cells and make them free a lot of weight, yet they'll adequately get undying all the while.

The diet is separated into three phases as clarified here, yet to sum things up: The "Hyper Success Phase" (motivated naming their folks), whereby dieters are limited to 1000kcals every day made up of three Sirtfood green juices and a sirtfood rich dinner. For three days in a row. Stage two then gets an extra 500kcal, on the grounds that you dump one of the juices and supplant it with real nourishment — Sirtfoods, however. Recollect that, it's significant. Toward the week's end, you go into the support period of 3 sirtfood rich dinners in addition to a Sirtfood juice.

The creators put this diet under a magnifying glass in their first class, private individual's rec center, where members (n=40) got instructional courses with a fitness coach and were under the creators' master healthful direction. They paid around £1,500 for the benefit as well. I think we'd all concur this was a thorough and replicable examination.

WHY IS SIRTFOOD DIET GOOD FOR YOU?

Benefits

The Sirtfood Diet depends on a new collection of foods called Sirtfoods. These wonderful nutrients in the body will activate an impressive reuse cycle that eliminates cellular waste and absorbs fat. Everything they do take our Sirtuine properties also called "thin" conditions. These are similar properties applied by exercise and fasting.

Top Sirtfoods Incorporate

PECANS	GREEN TEA	RED ONIONS	COCOA
PARSLEY	ADDITIONAL VIRGIN OLIVE OIL	STRAW-BERRY	CURRY FLAVORS
ESPRESSO	KALE	ROCKET	

Unlike recent advanced diets where the emphasis is on nutrition elimination, with Sirtfoods, the benefits are given by eating.

Preliminary members in our Sirtfood Diet lost an amazing 7 pounds over the underlying seven days, remembering increments for muscle and muscle work. This dramatic impact on fat-consuming, while muscle progression, is one reason that our Sirtfood-based Diet has gotten so well-known to anybody needing to get slender and fit as a fiddle, much the same as the world-class competitors and models. They have supported this way of eating. Alongside fat consuming, Sirtfoods additionally have one of some kind capacities to usually satisfy a craving, making them the ideal answer for accomplishing a healthy weight and supporting it long haul.

However, to consider it absolutely as a weight reduction diet is to overlook the main issue. This is a diet that has a lot to do with wellbeing as waistlines. Expanded vitality, brighter skin, feeling alarmed progressively, and better rest is the beautiful 'reactions' from along these lines of eating. Once in a while, the advantages are significantly increasingly momentous; remembering situations where following the diet for the more extended term has turned around metabolic ailments. Such is their health improving impacts that reviews demonstrate them to be all the more remarkable, then physician recommended tranquilizes in forestalling constant sickness, with benefits in diabetes, coronary illness, and Alzheimer's to give some examples. It's no big surprise that it is entrenched that the way of life eating the most Sirtfoods has been the least fatty and healthiest on the planet.

The main concern is evident: If you need to accomplish a progressively vivacious, slenderer, and healthier body, and establish the frameworks for deep-rooted health and protection from the ailment, at that point, the Sirtfood Diet is for you.

Can You Eat Meat On Sirtfood?

The diet plan does not just incorporates expending a good part of the meat; it suggests that protein be a primary consideration in a Sirtfood-based diet to receive the greatest reward in keeping up digestion and reducing the muscle exhaustion necessary in most diet plans. It is anything but a meat-overwhelming food (we despite everything recall the terrible breath from the Atkins diet), it's in reality very veggie lover well-disposed and caters for practically everybody, which is the thing that makes it so reasonable an alternative.

Leucine is an amino corrosive found in protein, which supplements and improves the activities of Sirtfoods. This implies the ideal approach to eating Sirtfoods is by consolidating them with a chicken breast, steak or another wellspring of leucine, for example, fish or eggs.

Poultry can be eaten uninhibitedly (because it is an excellent wellspring of protein, B nutrients, potassium and phosphorous). That red meat (another fantastic wellspring of protein, iron, zinc and nutrient B12) can be eaten up to multiple times (750g crude weight) seven days.

"Sirtfood" seems like something created by outsiders, brought to earth for human utilization with expectations of picking up mind control and global control. Sirt foods are foods high in sirtuins. Uh, come back once more? Sirtuins are a sort of protein that reviews on organic product flies, and mice have demonstrated direct digestion, increment bulk, and consume fat.

How Can It Work?

At its center, the way to getting in shape is genuinely straightforward: Create a calorie shortfall either by expanding your calorie consume exercises or diminishing your caloric admission. As it may, imagine a scenario where you could skirt the abstaining from excessive food intake and instead activate a "thin quality" without the requirement for extreme calorie limitation. This is the reason of The Sirtfood Diet, composed by nourishment specialists Aidan Goggin's and Glen Matten. The best approach to do it, they contend, is Sirt foods.

Sirtfoods are wealthy in supplements that activate an alleged "thin quality" called sirtuin. As indicated by Goggin's and Matten, the "thin quality" is activated when a lack of vitality is made after you confine calories. Sirtuins got fascinating to the nourishment world in 2003 when analysts found that resveratrol, a compound found in red wine, had a similar impact on life length as calorie limitation, however, it was accomplished without lessening admission. (Discover the complete truth about wine and its medical advantages.)

In the 2015 pilot study, testing the adequacy of sirtuins, the 39 members lost a normal of seven pounds in seven days. Those outcomes sound amazing. However, it's critical to understand this is a small example size concentrated over a brief timeframe. Weight reduction specialists additionally have their questions about the grandiose guarantees. The cases made are extremely theoretical and extrapolate from considers which were, for the most part, centered on basic creatures (like yeast) at the cell level. What occurs at the cell level doesn't mean what occurs in the human body at the full-scale level?

What Are the Advantages?

You will get thinner if you follow this eating regimen intently. Regardless of whether you're eating 1,000 calories of tacos, 1,000 calories of kale, or 1,000 calories of snicker doodles, you will get in shape at 1,000 calories. In any case, she likewise brings up that you can have accomplishments an increasingly sensible·calorie limitation. The typical day by day caloric admission of somebody not on a careful nutritional plan is 2,000 to 2,200, so diminishing to 1,500 is as yet confining and would be a viable weight reduction procedure for most.

Medical Advantages of Sirtfood Diet

Sirtfood diet diminishes the danger of heart infections, heftiness, diabetes, and early demise. Individuals who are following this eating regimen plan have encountered a few medical advantages, generally safe of ailment and prosperity. A portion of the regular medical advantages of sirtfood counts calories are as per the following:

It will assist you with losing fat, not muscles.

The eating routine won't deplete your vitality and rather keep you increasingly lively.

As it thoroughly relies upon diet, setting off to the rec center or performing thorough activities is a bit much.

The eating regimen plan stays away from the self-starvation hypothesis for weight reduction.

It forestalls various ceaseless illnesses as the nourishments remembered for this eating regimen plan are solid and nutritive.

Who Should Try Sirtfood Diet?

You know that you have overindulged during the holidays, but as you weigh yourself, you literally would want to shave all the extra pounds because you did not expect to have gained that much weight!

There is an upcoming wedding event, and you need to lose those extra pounds in order to fit yourself into your gown/suit. There is no way that you will lose that much weight in 2 months!

You know that you are overweight and just plain unhealthy. You have already tried a number of diets but to no avail. Either you feel that those diets are too restrictive, there is an adverse health effect, and the diet is too expensive to maintain. Speaking of maintenance, you have a hard time to keep off the little weight that you have managed to lose!

You are getting older, and you start to notice that aside from having a hard time dealing with hangovers and late-night parties, losing and maintaining weight is not that easy as it used to be. You are not a big fan of eliminating numerous food groups and doing rigorous exercise.

You have probably heard these scenarios too many times before, and you have probably experienced one or two or you are in one of these scenarios right now. Being overweight or obese is actually one of the most common health problems around the world. According to the world health organization, being overweight is when your BMI is equal to or greater than 25, while being obese is when you're BMI is equal to or greater than 30 (you can check your BMI here).

In the 2014 data from whom, worldwide obesity has more than doubled since 1980, and more than 1.9 billion adults are overweight; and it would be safe to conclude that after two years that that number has already increased significantly.

Health experts agree that this is a very alarming rate, but the good news is, obesity or having excess weight is preventable and reversible.

As you will notice, most of these scenarios are focused on the aesthetics – looking good and feeling more confident about your body, but what I would like to stress is the ill-effects of every extra bulge or pound that we carry. The possible health illnesses associated with being overweight is the primary reason why you need to try the revolutionary sirtfood diet.

SIRTFOOD TO ALWAYS EAT

Red Onion

Red onion has the most elevated centralization of quercetin, which enacts sirtuin. Yellow onion likewise contains noteworthy amounts. It is critical to eat them crude, to keep the degrees of supplements unaltered: truth be told, singed onions lose as much as 20% of quercetin during the procedure, a rate that arrives at 65% whenever cooked in the microwave and 75% whenever bubbled.

Onion contains a ton of water and has a decent measure of fructose sugar, which, notwithstanding giving it a specific pleasantness, gives it a mellow vitality work. Proteins and lipids are insignificant; cholesterol is missing. As to minerals and nutrients, there are no fixations deserving of specific note, so it is conceivable to state that the onion contains "a smidgen of everything."

Onion is appropriate for most food systems and, because of the substance of some somewhat zesty atoms, it tends to be contraindicated if there should be an occurrence of extreme touchiness and/or gastro-intestinal sicknesses, for example, stomach corrosive, gastritis, ulcer, peevish colon, hemorrhoids and gaps butt-centric. It has no contraindications for overweight and substitution pathologies; in actuality, it appears to apply a great effect on certain metabolic issues (hypertension, hypercholesterolemia).

The genuine "wealth" of this vegetable doesn't lie in the fiery, plastic, nutrient or saline supplements, yet in the phytotherapic particles (the majority of which have a cancer prevention agent and valuable capacity for the digestion). It doesn't contain gluten and lactose, and is acknowledged by veggie lover and vegetarian methods of reasoning. The normal part of the onion can arrive at 200 g (80 kcal).

Red Wine

Red wine is perfect for getting in shape and fat on the stomach because of its high substance of resveratrol, a substance that enacts sirtuins. Perfect to enjoy close to a large portion of a glass for every feast, better whenever joined by the other super nourishments sirt.

For the most part, when we talk about the advantages identified with the utilization of red wine, the primary particle that strikes a chord is resveratrol (on which there are many affirmed logical investigations).

Metabolic properties of cancer prevention agent, antibacterial, antifungal, hostile to the tumor, mitigating and blood fluidization properties are ascribed to this non-flavonoid phenol. Under specific conditions, one glass of red wine every day could decrease the rate of cluster related stroke by up to half. Most likely, it is because of resveratrol and different polyphenols that the purported "French Paradox" happens: During the 1980s, some epidemiological investigations rose that — in spite of the bounty of soaked unsaturated fats and cholesterol in the eating routine — in France, the frequency of hypercholesterolemia and cardiovascular pathologies was lower than in other dietetically equivalent nations.

It was guessed on this evident conundrum that the utilization of red wine could secure against coronary illness; today, such proof has been emphatically addressed. Resveratrol likewise seems to shield the cerebrum from subjective decrease identified with Alzheimer's malady.

As of late, by dissecting the arrangement of red wine, researchers from the "College of California at Davis" found another gathering of atoms fit for battling overabundance blood cholesterol. These are saponins, or liquor solvent frothing substances that are equipped for restricting cholesterol in the digestive system (counting that of bile salts), lessening their retention. An examination by the "Oregon States College of Agricultural Studies"

has rather watched the response of guinea pigs to a nourishing system wealthy in fats, with and without red wine extricates. All mice indicated the equivalent metabolic outcomes average of overweight stationary people, however, those who took care of red wine remove uncovered less amassing of fat in the liver and lower glucose levels.

The atom liable for this response would be ellagic corrosive (likewise present in numerous vegetables and natural products, for example, pomegranate), or a phenolic cancer prevention agent equipped for forestalling the gathering of fat in the phones and restricting the advancement of new adipocytes. As though that were insufficient, red wine is additionally rich in quercetin. This flavonoid (tetraoxyflavonol) speaks to a metabolic inhibitor of certain catalysts associated with the provocative reaction. The cancer prevention agent elements of quercetin are to reestablish tocopherols (vit. E), detoxify cells from superoxide, and reduction the emission of nitric oxide during irritation. Besides, as indicated by the American Cancer Society, this flavonoid goes about as an amazing anticancer, particularly in the colon.

Red wine is rich in supposed tannins, otherwise called proanthocyanidins; these phenolic mixes, liable for the red shade, are exceptionally renowned for their potential gainful activity at the cardiovascular level.

Espresso

Espresso additionally contains sirtuins, which permit you to consume fat and dispose of additional pounds. Drink a limit of 3 cups every day, better without sugar to not surpass the calories.

Among the numerous nourishing segments of espresso, the most popular and most contemplated is without a doubt caffeine, as it has significant properties, for example:

The stimulatory impact on gastric and biliary emissions (which is the reason an espresso toward the finish of the supper is accepted to encourage processing).

The tonic and invigorating impact on cardiovascular and anxious capacity (this is the reason numerous individuals value its vivacious impact, which is helpful, in addition to other things, so as not to bum after a healthy dinner).

The lipolytic impact, that is, the thinning help (caffeine invigorates the utilization of fats for vitality and thermogenesis, expanding the quantity of calories consumed by the "human machine").

The anorectic impact (espresso taken in monstrous dosages diminishes hunger).

Notwithstanding caffeine, there are numerous substances in espresso, the potential useful job of which on the body is still under investigation. Specifically, a few segments have been disengaged with solid cancer prevention agent, against mutagenic and mitigating properties, which are anyway deficient to make up for the hazard getting from high utilization of espresso.

Cabbage

Cabbage: this vegetable flaunts enormous amounts of quercetin and kaempferol, which initiate sirtuin. It is additionally an extremely normal and simple to discover vegetable, just as being modest.

As a matter of first importance, cabbage speaks to a legitimate regular calming: On account of the amount of mineral salts and nutrients of which it is created, cabbage assumes the job of immaculate detoxifier and can kill poisons, along these lines speaking to a solid anticancer food, particularly against specific kinds of malignant growth, including bosom, colon and bladder. Continuously for similar reasons, it fortifies the safe framework and goes about as a blazing if there should arise an occurrence of infections and diseases of different sorts.

Because of the huge number of flavonoids present in it, cabbage assists with forestalling untimely maturing and to act against free radicals. However, not just! The nearness of fiber controls absorption and intestinal action, just as a right working of the heart. Truth be told, on account of the amino acids of which it is rich, cabbage adds to keeping the weight low, speaking to a substantial guide against hypertension.

Cabbages are a valuable goods of nutrient C, folic corrosive, which can animate the safe framework, just as fiber, potassium. They additionally contain substances, for example, thiooxazolidones, with a subterranean insect thyroid impact, and sulforaphane, which, joined with isothiocyanates, is accepted to have a defensive impact against intestinal tumors.

They are very satisfying nourishments and thusly are exceptionally helpful in a low-calorie diet. Cabbages play out a valuable detoxifying activity for the body and are a ground-breaking calming; they are especially shown if there should be an occurrence of frailty, abscesses, cystitis, and gastric ulcers.

Bean Stew Pepper

Bean stew is a vegetable utilized essentially as a zest, new or dry. In different nations, for instance, in Central and South America, on account of the propensity for the fiery taste, enormous amounts of bean stew are eaten each day.

Bean stew peppers have a moderate vitality consumption, predominantly gave via sugars (fructose); proteins are scant, as are lipids.

It is sans cholesterol and contains a decent level of dietary fiber.

Ready bean stew is especially plentiful in nutrients; the substance in ascorbic corrosive is especially applicable (229mg of nutrient C per 100 grams of new organic product). Likewise, vital is the liberal nearness of carotenoids (forerunners of nutrient an) and a moderate grouping of niacin (or nutrient PP).

The admission of mineral salts, particularly potassium, is likewise acceptable; the degrees of calcium and phosphorus are less intriguing, however important.

This bright arrangement of dietary standards (except for nutrient C), is additionally amassed in the zest pepper, at that point in the dried and perhaps powdered organic product; similarly, the zesty flavor with which consistently is given a little panache to the blander dishes is likewise reinforced.

The most extravagant bean stew pepper is the Thai one, to be utilized to make each dish delectable and reactivate the digestion. Add it to first courses, second courses, and vegetable soups and… indeed, even chocolate!

Chocolate

Talking about chocolate, uplifting news! It isn't just acceptable, yet in addition, wealthy in flavonoids, substances that initiate sirtuins. You can eat up to three squares every day to top off on cancer prevention agents and get in shape, battling the feeling of yearning. Better to pick the dull one to restrict calories!

On the off chance that the facts confirm that the best nourishments are additionally the most hazardous for wellbeing, chocolate is by all accounts the great exemption that affirms the standard in any event to some degree.

Dim chocolate, because of its cocoa content, speaks to one of the most liberal food wellsprings of flavonoids, eminent cancer prevention agents present in nourishments of root or plant beginning, for example, tea, red wine, citrus products of the soil.

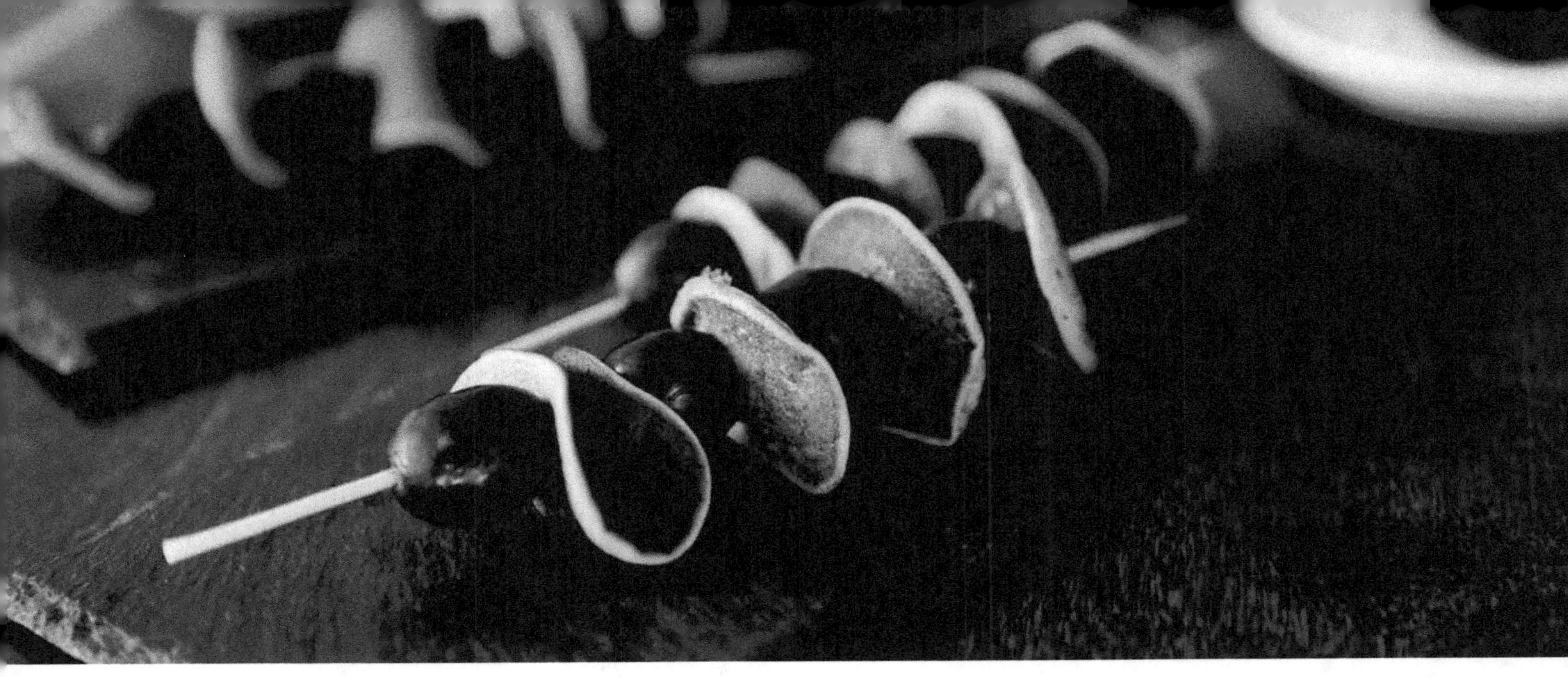

CONCLUSION

Thank you for making it to the end. It's true that 6 out of every 10 Americans are currently struggling to live their lives through the pain and discomfort of the disease, but these statistics don't have to keep declining. You now have enough knowledge to make lifestyle changes that are going to protect you from being on the wrong end of these statistics.

Despite the incredible advances that science has made in the fields of health, the body, and medicine, our world is getting sicker by the day. I am sure that part of this reason is that this knowledge is being passed around only by an elite few doctors, researchers and dieticians. The more you know about your own body, the more power is in your own control to protect your health.

It doesn't matter where your health is right now. What matters is what you're going to do about it from now on. You know you need to change and, hopefully, you now have a good foundation in some simple, effective and relatively enjoyable ways you can change your health for the better.

Actively Advocate for Your Own Health

This book was written to be much more than just another diet book. The goal was to spark excitement and interest in your heart about your own health. Too many of us go through our lives assuming that we should not be held responsible for our health—that is the realm of doctors and professional healers.

But the more you can learn about how your body operates, the better equipped you will be to take control of your own health, rather than waiting for it to deteriorate to the point where you need a doctor's intervention.

The human body is a remarkable machine. It is designed with a more advanced natural defense system than current medical science even fully understands. The amount we do know, however, tells us that in order for these natural defenses to effectively protect us from disease, they need 2 things: energy and nutrition.

Those components also need to be well balanced, as too much or too little energy can throw the entire system off balance.

The 21st century has given us an incredible bounty of food, so we have all the energy and nutrition available to us easily, without being forced to hunt it down for ourselves as our ancestors did.

Unfortunately, we also have an abundance of new foods available to us. Foods that over-deliver on the first requirement, energy, and under-deliver on the second requirement, nutrition. Knowing this, we can work towards finding the right balance once again.

With every additional nutrient-dense sirtuin-activating food source you consume, you are proactively working towards rebalancing those scales.

Continue Moving Forward! The Sirtfood Diet is not a temporary or quick fix, but it is a lifestyle that you can adopt to prioritize your health for the rest of your life.

Temporary weight loss followed by a sustained weight gain is the way of calorie restricting, time-bound diets. They're unpleasant to follow, often require a lot of math and calculations, and they are not serving you.

Diets that are rich in delicious and health-supporting nutrition help your body optimize itself. The Sirtfood Diet isn't about restricting anything in your life. It's focused on all the good things you can add to feel great, look fantastic, and become the healthiest, best version of yourself at any age or stage in your life.

This book did not set out to give you a prescriptive diet blueprint to follow, planning out your every bite for you. Instead, the goal was to help you understand the value of the foods you choose to eat, so that you can learn how to make these choices for yourself, automatically and with full confidence.

Of course, it always helps to have a selection of choices to choose from, so now that you're ready to start this Sirtfood Diet for yourself

You're set to start living your best life, and you deserve to feel healthy, energetic and beautiful. To help you make these conditions of a great life a reality for you, the Sirtfood Diet is the last diet you will ever need.

Congratulations and Bon Appetit!